The Joy of Juice Fasting

The JOY of Juice Fasting

for
Health + Cleansing + Weight Loss

Klaus Kaufmann

Foreword by Luc DeShepper MD PhD

Vancouver
Canada

The Joy of Juice Fasting

Published by
alive books
P O Box 80055
Burnaby BC
Canada V5H 3X1

Copyright© 1990 by Klaus Kaufmann

Cover Photo: Siegfried Gursche
Back Cover Photo: Siegfried Gursche
Typesetting/layout: Robert W. Oates
Cover Design: Irene Hannestad

First printing — **December** 1990

Canadian Cataloguing in Publication Data

Kaufmann, Klaus, 1942 —
    The joy of juice fasting

ISBN 0-920470-22-X

    1. Fasting.   2. Fruit juice — Therapeutic use.
3. Vegetable juices — Therapeutic use..
    I Title.   II Author

RM226.5.K38 1990   613.2'6   C89-091471-0

Dedicated to better human health, and to my wife, Gabriele, without whose enthusiasm I would have been poorer in experience though "richer" in appearance

This book is informational only and should not be considered as a substitute for consultation with a duly-licensed medical doctor. Any attempt to diagnose and treat an illness should come under the direction of a physician. The author is not himself a medical doctor and does not purport to offer medical advice, make diagnoses, prescribe remedies for specific medical conditions or substitute for medical consultation.

Acknowledgments

People have waited a long time for this book to appear. Well, here it is. Of all those who extended a helping hand in the writing, I offer my deepest gratitude to my publisher, Siegfried Gursche. Siegfried gave me both the opportunity and the computer on which to store my research material over a four year period. The clarity of my endnotes is owed to Ingrid Wood, as is the inclusion of the keyword "joy" in the title which initially read "The Magic of Juice Fasting." Putting a book together on computer is in itself a difficult task as any experienced writer will vouchsafe. To explain the delay; there were hitches. At the time of writing *The Joy of Juice Fasting* I was simultaneously committing my other book, *Silica — The Forgotten Nutrient*, to computer memory. Retaining the two volumes proved to be an ordeal my IBM-clone just couldn't sustain — perhaps because it was still unpaid for! My computer somehow "lost" the entire "electronic" manuscript of this present work in its convoluted memory banks, leaving me with the chore of rewriting the whole book from memory (with the help of Ginko Biloba!). Oh well, what are writers for? The loving support of my wife, Gabriele, resulted in her active participation in this book, as detailed elsewhere. The Hermann Hesse poem was indirectly inspired by my friend Christina Druzinsky. Finally, the physical beauty of this work owes its existence to the dedicated efforts of Robert W. Oates and Irene Hannestad.

The Joy of Juice Fasting is:

- Stimulating + Rejuvenating

- The Healthiest Approach To Cleansing + Healing

- A Natural Protection Against Disease

- A Way To Lose Pounds + Gain Admiration

- A Source of Energy + A Purifier of Body + Mind

- Prevents Premature Aging

- Not Another Fad Diet

- A Way to Find Out Why, When and How to Juice Fast

- How To Break Your Juice Fast

- Being Aware of What To Avoid

Contents

Foreword

If it would depend on the number of books and pamphlets written by physicians, nutritionists and physical fitness buffs, we all would be slender and beautiful. How is it then, that not all of us are? It is definitely not because of a lack of reading material. Looking healthy, svelte and radiant is a dream chased by most people on this planet. Therefore, every new "fenomenal" diet appearing on the market becomes a way of life for many — at least for a while. Many are willing to spend a small fortune on a pill that promises slender bodies without any effort. And yet, Mother Nature provides us with the best introduction to any diet: fasting. This word is not going to win any popularity contest with most of the people. Pictures of starving people, calamities of dryness, earthquakes and tornado's creating food shortness, flash through our minds. Why should anybody in their right mind want to do this on a voluntary basis? And yet, fasting has proven to be one of the most efficient healers in history. In ancient cultures, fasting periods of up to fourteen days were incorporated BEFORE medicine was given, preparing the patient for a maximum effect of the plant extract. Of course, we don't have to go that far, all of us have done some fasting in life; our first reflex when we are sick is to fast or at least reduce food intake.

This book is an excellent guide to convince anybody

who wants to create happiness and health in a relatively short time. A three day fast leads to increased energy, enhanced perception and often gives the patient his first glimpse of true well-being. In case you are still convinced that fasting is not for you (it is probably the compulsive eater in you who suggests this), the first chapters of this work explain in simple lay-person's terms why juice fasting is for everyone. Every possible question about each facet of fasting is anticipated and answered. No matter in what stage of health or disease you are, juice fasting can be introduced and this book teaches you how!

Luc DeSchepper MD PhD

Everyone can be magical
Everyone can reach his goals
if he can think
if he can wait
if he can fast

Hermann Hesse

Translated from the German by Klaus Kaufmann

Introduction

This is not a diet book! The world doesn't need another diet book. Too many fad diet books have already been published, and too many have as their underlying aim the promotion of expensive diet products that are themselves often of dubious value. It's of the utmost importance to distinguish the concept of fasting from that of dieting. Fasting is neither fad nor diet. Maybe the reason dieticians don't advocate fasting is that to do so could put them out of a job? Chances are that the people who most vehemently warn against fasting have never fasted, but experts will tell you that eating and not eating are comparable to waking and sleeping; two mutually beneficial states. Actually everybody is familiar with fasting. We don't eat when asleep, hence the first meal of the day is called breakfast.

The ancient art of fasting is revolutionized by the new concept of *juice fasting* as expounded in this book. A fresh approach to fasting, it can be of the greatest benefit to both healthy and sick, both overweight or slim people alike. But fasting is much more than weight reduction; it opens the gates to rejuvenation and a healthier and happier life.

By granting the metabolism some time off from its heavy workload, fasting makes manifest the purifying nature of the organism in the absence of solid food, and

1

its own benefits to the body as a whole. The result of isolation and subsequent union puts the conscious thinking mind in harmony with the subconscious mind which controls the physical processes. It connects the personal life of the individual to the forces of nature, thus regenerating overall balance. In this way juice fasting results in weight reduction, health restoration, and spiritual renewal. After a juice fast, the individual emerges one step closer to being that perfectly poised human being.

You may have been searching for a practical guide to fasting when you reached for this book, weighing the juice fasting alternative in your own mind. I trust the guidelines given will help to strengthen your resolution and bring you a step closer to a new and joyful reality. A day-by-day account of my own and my wife's juice fasting adventure follows and details both our losses and gains.

Juice fasting can be approached in a variety of ways. You can easily create recipe modifications best suited to your personal requirements, choosing for yourself the appropriate juice and the best fast for your particular circumstances. Juice fasting is exactly what its name suggests; fasting! However, while fasting you are provided with delicious-tasting liquids and nourishment, while still giving your digestion the much-needed rest. The joy of juice fasting is the newest discovery at exclusive Continental health spas. In most English-speaking countries it is quickly becoming a popular approach to weight control, cleansing, healing, and a new spiritualism. As the title suggests, juice fasting truly can be seen as joy and is pure magic.

I have included appetizing recipes that permit actual feasting during fasting, together with step-by-step instructions on how to prepare for and how to proceed during a juice fast. Frankly, fasting can be a treat. You can feel stimulated, elated. It is easy to maintain a sunny disposition throughout a juice fast. On completion you will feel proud of your successes, content in the knowledge that you have accomplished a great deal — more than most people ever dream of!

An *internal juice fasting rinse* flushes your body clean. It is far easier to adapt to than any diet, not least because you will not feel hungry during a juice fast. Because you are drinking juice, easily transported in a thermos bottle to just about anywhere, you can fit juice fasting into your regular routines at home, at work or while travelling. There is no fussing with complicated food preparations or purchasing of expensive ingredients. The necessary arrangements for juice fasting are incredibly simple.

Juice fasting is also the gentlest route to weight loss. It bypasses the "starvation anxiety" caused by going completely without nourishment. Throughout the juice fast the body is continually provided with vital minerals, vitamins, and enzymes. The metabolism is not deprived of essential nutrients and can thrive on a rest from solid food.

It is common to lose 10 pounds of unwanted weight within one week. I did! The cleansing process activated by a juice fast normalizes cholesterol and blood pressure levels while relieving both tension and insomnia. Juice fasting induces a natural high and increases the pleasure you gain from your after-fast-meals. It helps slow the aging process; you actually feel younger. It trains you not to overeat. Juice fasting eliminates toxins from the body and your new condition can be a great help towards giving up smoking, alcohol or other drugs, although ideally you should have these things out of your life completely even before undertaking a juice fast.

The main purpose of this book is to introduce the concept and the delights of juice fasting, but the healing powers of juice fasting therapy offer new hope also to those in need of health restoration. Our ancestors used fasting as a restorative treatment before modern civilization obscured their innate wisdom. It is well known that animals in the wild, without the services of a veterinarian, utilize fasting as a natural method to cure their ills. Even my own pet will "go on a fast," refusing to eat from time to time. Often it heals its ailment before there is a need to visit the vet, since, like many pets, it hates the trip to the veterinary clinic.

1

Juice Alone!

The Safest and Most Effective Reducing Method Known

Fasting with the addition of just juice leads to improved dietary habits and is, as I will show, absolutely safe. Overeating, on the other hand, is harmful to the body and at times has even lead to death. Fortunately, it is possible to shed the extra pounds through juice fasting. The juice fasting method offers a safe approach to weight loss, while many fasting methods fail to make adequate provisions for a supply of essential vitamins, minerals and enzymes. A lot of fasting experts advocate total abstention, allowing just distilled water. Some fasts even fail to consider an adequate supply of liquids, but while the human body is able to live without solid food for weeks, maybe months, it cannot go without fluids for longer than three days. There are "fasting gurus" who recommend drinking only water during a fast. Some advocate enemas during fasting while others are totally opposed to enemas. There are those who suggest complete bed rest and others who advocate regular exercise during the fast. The multitude of books on the subject are baffling with contradictory claims. There is much confusion surrounding the subject of fasting. With so much seemingly paradoxical advice, it's no wonder that a person becomes perplexed searching for the proper fasting method. A practical approach, though, can avoid all problems.

Before you fast, ask yourself some questions. What are your reasons for undertaking a fast? Do you want to reduce your weight? Do you want to prevent or heal an illness? Do you want to prevent premature aging? Do you want to cleanse your system? Are you hoping for insight into your own functions? If you answered yes to any or all of these questions, then fasting is for you. Juice fasting can help accomplish all these goals. Old as it is, fasting can be seen as a modern, scientific health-restoring and rejuvenating miracle. Not only does it accomplish physiological regeneration, it revitalizes the body. In doing so, the fast helps sharpen mental acuity, aesthetic perception and increases spiritual awareness.

Many of the constantly advertised fad and reducing diets are actually harmful to the system. This cannot be said of juice fasting. Not only will you be able to reduce safely, on the average one pound per day, you will in fact improve your health while reducing. Instead of experimenting with questionable reducing diets, try juice fasting. There are many benefits.

Fasting is one of the oldest therapies known to man. We instinctively stop eating when we are feeling ill and abstain from food until our health is restored. Hippocrates, the ancient father of medicine, prescribed fasting. So did the famed Paracelsus, the first allopath who called fasting "the greatest remedy; the physician within." Frequent fasting is habitually taken advantage of by religious leaders. Fasting increases mental efficiency, leads to more acute perception and helps to increase longevity.

Modern medicine, with its penchant for prescribing artificial drugs, has seemingly forgotten the simple healing available at low or even no cost. The strong, artificial drugs that are often prescribed as aids in fasting, include health-destroying amphetamines. These definitely, undeniably, lead the body towards disease and destruction.

Fortunately, changes are occurring for the better. People are beginning to appreciate again that it's perfectly OK to fast. Why was fasting forgotten for so long? No one knows, but the advantages of fasting were never altogether lost. The Bible[1], for instance, supports fasting for a great many psychological, philosophical and practical reasons. The Good Book describes fasting as "abstaining from physical nourishment," and proves its capability to heal private afflictions, grief, anxiety. We are told that Jesus fasted 40 days and 40 nights! Other spiritual books contain similar references to fasting.

Today, medical circles are again recognizing the healing powers of fasting. One of the greatest fasting specialists in Germany, Prof. Dr. Werner Zabel, proclaimed, "Together with fever and optimal nutrition, fasting is man's oldest and best healing method."[2] He is absolutely right, the therapeutic effect of fasting is indeed well documented.

The well-known Canadian physician, Hans Selye, M.D., says, "Life, the biological chain that holds our parts together, is only as strong as the weakest vital link.[3]" Once you understand that each cell of your body is a complete living entity in its own right, having its own metabolism, you can begin to understand this statement. It is truly sad that people mistreat their body cells, and for years disrespect their bodily processes. Many attempt to cure mental anguishes with overeating, and then, to make matters worse, consume foods that are neither nutritious nor wholesome.

Despite constant abuse over a very long time, the cells faithfully perform. They work around the clock and around the toxins bombarding the metabolism. The cells most carefully separate the good from the bad and, as much as possible, eliminate toxins and waste. But when there is a continuous overflow of food, the battered body succumbs at long last to the constant onslaught of too much, overly rich, over-abundant, nutritionally poor food. At this point the weakened cells start to lose their ability to change surplus nutrients into lipids, or fats, and to deposit these "relatively" safe items into fat tissues for storage and possible later breakdown, such as occurs with fasting. Overtaxed, the body's system reaches a deadlock. The multitude of toxins can no longer be properly eliminated or dealt with by an overworked metabolism. A point is quickly reached when toxic wastes are accumulated in various tissues, especially bone tissue. Eventually the cells break down from overload, the body retaliates against its occupant. The occupant, the person, becomes ill.

Too often it is only then that the sufferer begins to wonder, "Why am I suddenly sick? What is the cause?" But just how sudden was the approach of illness? For how many uncounted years did the body silently do its best and not complain? And how often did the stricken person override minor symptoms? "Oh, the headache will pass, the pain will go away, swallow painkillers for it." The pain killed, the body seemingly kept on performing dutifully and quietly. But the day of reckoning came eventually. At whose expense?

Juice fasting can give your body a much-needed break and give it a chance to eliminate the accumulated toxins and reduce the overabundance of lipids. Proper juice fasting allows the body to continue to function normally while repairing itself. By ridding your body of dead and useless cells, you are stimulating the construction and growth of new, fresh, healthy cells, you are literally *rejuvenating* yourself.

During a prolonged fast, within the first three days, the body will begin to live off its own substance. Deprived of needed nutrients, particularly protein and fats, it burns and digests its own tissues. But it doesn't do this indiscriminately. It very carefully selects first of all your diseased, damaged, aged and dead cells. In its innate wisdom, your body feeds on all the impurities, toxins, fats and waste materials it was forced to build up over a long period of time.

Every good gardener knows that once in a while there is a need to burn the piled-up refuse heap. After three days of fasting, your body begins to burn off its rubbish, while maintaining and even revitalizing its essential tissues and organs, glands, nerves and the brain. It has been observed that the protein level in the blood stream of fasting people remained constant and normal throughout the fasting period, even though no protein was consumed.*

During a juice fast, the cleansing capacity of the evacuatory organs — lungs, liver, kidneys, and skin — is greatly increased, while masses of toxins are quickly expelled. During fasting, the level of toxins in the urine can be ten times higher than normal because the kidneys are being freed of the burden of dealing with constantly accumulating poisons that are found in various ingested food particles. A juice fast affords a physiological rest to your digestive system. Fresh vegetable or fruit juices, carefully selected for purity, require very little digestion and are easily assimilated by the upper digestive tract without putting any burden on the digestive organs. Following a juice fast, your digestion is greatly improved, the rejuvenated cells find it easier to deal with nutrients and oxygen more efficiently, therefore sluggishness and waste retention are prevented.

* *Research by the Second Medical University Clinic of Hamburg, Eppendorf, Germany*

2

Healing Juice Therapy

Thomas A. Edison[4], who gave the world the first work-
able electric light bulb, has said: *"The doctor of the future
will give no medicine but will interest his patients in the care
of the human frame, in diet, and in the cause and prevention of
disease."* May all physicians always search for that light.

The German doctor and fasting specialist, Otto H. F.
Buchinger, M.D.[5], stated that there are basically two main
groups of diseases — those in which one *must* fast and
those in which one *may* fast. The *"must"* relates to actual
manifested diseases, the *"may"* to the prevention of diseases. Preventive voluntary fasting is obviously prefer-
able to curative mandatory fasting.

One in Ten
Controlled fasting in the treatment of serious diseases is
recommended by a number of medical experts, notably
by Dr. Buchinger, M.D., and should only be undertaken
with medical supervision. "Controlled juice fasting is the
best therapy to glowing health," says the famous Austrian
naturopathic expert Rudolph Breuss[6] who advocates juice
fasting for numerous ailments and diseases. He even recommends controlled juice fasting as an effective cancer
treatment. Rudolph Breuss prescribes a forty-two day
medically supervised juice fast as an initial treatment for
cancer.

Most people never fast and may never do so. They consider it unhealthy. They are wrong. Benjamin Franklin is credited with the seemingly mystical words: "Nine men in ten are suicides[7]." It seems he meant that people who do not make a conscious effort to retain their health do commit suicide after a fashion. There is a warning here that continuous intoxication, the taking in of toxins, is deadly. Increasingly we are being offered all the wrong foods and an astounding ninety percent of the population (Franklin's figures are mathematically "right on.") eat them unquestioningly. *Only one person out of ten follows a healthful diet.* Such dire statistics confirm the urgent need for change.

Just the other day I heard on the news that, in our big cities, breathing itself is dangerous because accumulated toxins in the air cannot escape during a heat wave. In the absence of a relieving wind factor people are actually advised to escape metropolitan areas if they can! Our world is increasingly being poisoned. The skies are constantly polluted by airplanes, smoke-stacks, and an ever increasing amount of automotive exhaust, all pumping tons of deadly toxins into the atmosphere. No wonder that there is such a huge hole in the earth's ozone layer that scientists on a recent North Pole expedition got severe sunburn. Humankind is playing a dangerous game with Mother Nature.

Our waterways, lakes and rivers are equally polluted. Powerful chemical disinfectants, mainly chlorine, are used to make water "drinkable," and crops are sprayed with pesticides and insecticides to increase net yield of seed and fruit. But little food value is left in such seeds and fruits. The chemicals used are meant to kill off pests only but the residues remain and reach us through the foods we ingest. Nowadays we even have to contend with radioactive fallout, the most pernicious poison, because of its extensive half-life. Such effects as those of Three Mile Island and the Chernobyl nuclear disasters are almost impossible to rectify.

Synthetic additives dumped into edible foods are another cause for concern. Meat products in particular are regularly impregnated with harmful substances designed to make naturally quick-spoiling meat last longer. Others are added to prevent discoloration and impart flavor thereby boosting purchase appeal.

All these poisons enter the bloodstream, cause havoc and damage the health. A properly conducted juice fast can aid in freeing the blood of all accumulated deadly poisons.

Acidosis is an imbalance of the blood; a condition that is characterized by hyperacidity, with an acid-alkali balance (ph-value) of less than seven. It is evident in a wide variety of symptoms, including headaches, skin eruptions, and the common cold, but can be easily corrected. A healthy acid-alkaline balance in the blood can be re-established by avoiding acid-forming foods and by providing alkaline-forming nourishment instead. This can be accomplished through juice fasting because raw vegetable and fruit juices are alkaline-forming. Re-establishment of the acid-alkaline balance can be hastened by the ingestion of L(+) lactic acid fermented juices*.

Perhaps you are one of those people who are afflicted by a variety of symptoms but have been unable to find the right doctor or treatment for your illness? Don't give up hope. Juice fasting is worth your earnest consideration.

If it is true that we unknowingly contribute to the

---

* *An excellent, easy-to-understand account of the health promoting power of L(+) lactic acid can be found in Chapter ix, page 162, of the book "How to Fight Cancer & Win" by William L. Fischer, published by alive books, 1988*

cause of our own illnesses through the continued neglect of our environment, while equally neglecting body, mind and spirit, then why are certain people predisposed to disease while others seem to get away unscathed? It may very well be true that disease causing agents have lodged inside the body because the *"predisposed"* have unkowningly or carelessly ingested them with their food. According to one of the world's leading nutritionists, the late Dr. Paavo Airola, N.D., Ph.D.[8], the body tends to deposit toxins that can no longer be properly eliminated due to an oversupply of food. These enter the bone tissue in the form of crystals, eventually causing joint ailments.

It's discouraging that few people are actively pursuing their health by practicing disease prevention. Most pay attention to their health only when it is too late, when disease has struck. Then too often they look for the "quick fix." Instead of just blaming it on *predisposition* to one illness or another, they could well be able to heal themselves with a supervised juice fast. If, on the other hand, they are truly genetically disadvantaged and predisposed to certain diseases and viral attacks, then it becomes imperative to maintain health through the regular cleansing of their inner and outer body environments.

Many authenticated reports exist on the healing and restorative effects of juice fasting. Nevertheless, each individual case is somewhat different and specific treatments must be adjusted to each person's needs. Mental and physical conditions must be taken into consideration before a medicinally-inspired juice fast is undertaken. I strongly recommend seeking the advice of a competent naturopathic physician before an attempt to heal specific diseases through juice fasting is undertaken.

Generally, though, in both chronic and less serious conditions, juice fasting therapy can be safely undertaken on your own, keeping in mind that fasting doesn't in itself effect a cure of any disease or illness. However, through fasting your invigorated body and mind are handed a "new license," new strength obtained from the purification of the system, to fight off disease and illness. Raw juices, in addition to their medicinal properties in the treatment of most diseases, purify the blood and all the body's tissues. Juice fasting has been used to heal a variety of conditions. Some ailments in which relief and even complete healing has been reported by reliable sources include:

Allergies, anemia, angina, arthritis, asthma, blood diseases, chronic lower back pain, chronic headaches, chronic constipation, chronic tonsillitis, chronic bronchitis, circulatory disorders, diabetes (under doctor control), eczema, emphysema, gall bladder inflammation, gastric catarrh, gastritis, goiter, gout, halitosis (bad breath), heart disease, high blood pressure, infections, insomnia, irregular heart beat, kidney diseases, leg ulcers, liver ailments, low blood pressure, nervousness, neuritis, obesity, overweight, polycythemia, prostate disorders, psoriasis, rheumatic disorders, skin disorders, sterility and stomach disorders.

Juice fasting can be used to trace the sources of food allergies. It has also been successful in treating some mental illness, like schizophrenia.

Juice fasting improves your sex life. From the fact that surplus body energy serves to stimulate sexual vigor it follows that a person in poor health makes a poor lover. When bodily functions are restored to normal, when pain is washed away by internal cleansing, a new vitality emerges. Sexual activity is one of the greatest joys that man and woman are blessed with. Lack of interest in sex can be a sign of poor health of body and mind, except, of course where abstinence is practiced for religious or personal reasons.

15

There are a few conditions where prolonged fasting is inadvisable, such as in advanced cases of tuberculosis, active malignancies, advanced diabetes, during pregnancy or breastfeeding, and in extreme cases of emaciation. Whenever there is a serious, acute disease process, fasting should not be attempted before consulting a doctor and abiding by that decision on the wisdom of undertaking a fast.

This equally applies to patients who are currently undergoing drug therapies like insulin, digitalis, cortisone, penicillin or any other strong drug. Coffee should be left alone when fasting even if you have been a heavy coffee drinker for years though this may lead to a headache after a 24 hour withdrawal period. The headache, if it arises, will vanish soon. Any drug withdrawal is best undertaken gradually during a juice fast, under the careful supervision of a physician.

What The Doctor Says About Juice Fasting[9]

"Fasting and sticking to the resolution of abstention is the renunciation of the overeating of solid food, usual in our everyday eating habits. At the same time, fasting represents a return to nature and natural ways which include fasting. Because a complete fast — the so-called zero-diet — results in a deficiency of minerals, vitamins and enzymes, such a momentous interference into the bodily processes should never be contemplated without consulting a physician.

Juice fasting, on the other hand, supplies liquid nourishment to the system. For the duration of the fast, the system is switched to a slower low-burning metabolism. During this time the organism is forced to live off its own substance, but thanks to the juice, is not deprived of vital regulatory vitamins, minerals and enzymes.

Among the beneficial effects are:

- A cleansing of your complete intestinal tract
- A conditioning of your digestion
- The mobilization of self-help measures of your organism
- The stimulation of your inner secretions
- The reduction of waste material deposits
- And the hastening of cell regeneration, effecting thereby a rejuvenation of your tissues and organs.

There are other benefits. The human organism requires protein for its maintenance work. When this is withheld, as during a juice fast, the reduction of excessive, mainly fatty, deposits begins. These deposits are now utilized by the body and, in effect, eaten, or changed into needed building blocks. The positive result becomes evident after a short time. The human being, in a oneness of body, mind and soul, feels freer and redeemed. The feeling of well-being becomes increased; those of physical freshness and greater mobility are beginning. Altogether this leads to an elevated mood in the fasting person. Such feelings are recorded time and again in fasting clinics. Finally, though this is not the primary goal of a limited juice fasting period, the body weight is toned down to a more natural level.

There are two recommended methods for juice fasting, a short eight day cleansing and rejuvenating fast or the full-sized two by six day vibrant reducing fast."

The Overweight Illness

Is obesity or being overweight truly a disease? To answer this question correctly, let's look at what causes excess weight. Dr. Buchinger[10] says, it is the result of:

1. A lazier elimination process in bowels, kidneys and skin due to reduced combustion in the metabolism.

2. The glands not performing properly. The pituitary, thyroid, adrenal glands and ovaries and testes have all been the cause of excess weight in chronically overweight people.

3. A faulty fat metabolism including disturbances of the body's water economy and assimilation problems.

Even though it is not a disease as such, obesity certainly seems to be an ailment. Dr. Buchinger notes[11] that as a physician he most frequently diagnoses both a disease and an overweight* problem, stating "high blood pressure *and* overweight, angina pectoris *and* overweight, severe rheumatism *and* overweight, skin and other diseases *and* overweight," et cetera as the patients ailment. He goes on to say that "the customary use of purgatives is not suitable for losing weight, but only for causing injury to the intestinal area, and the peristaltic movement, and for disturbing the calcium content of the blood."

And then he tells us, "It is easy to see that **health fasting** as a rather heroic method of treatment makes considerable demands on the intelligence, willpower and character of the fasting person. The healing fast alone can help towards getting well," concluding with "people with all types of obesity not only can but should fast! For the waste products and stores of fat are then broken down, burnt up and eliminated; and central disturbances (glands, water economy, etc.) are again regulated to normal

* *According to the Stanford Heart Disease Prevention Program you can calculate your "ideal" weight, simply, as follows: Females — height in inches x 3.5 lbs minus 108; Males — height in inches x 4.0 lbs minus 128. Large frame add 8%, small frame substract 4%*

healthy functions."

I suppose we can safely conclude that overweight has at least a "heavy hand" in becoming sick. However, in therapeutic juice fasting, aimed at healing existing ailments or preventing them, weight loss is of secondary importance and individual results should not be compared among persons. Weight reduction, or its absence, in therapeutic fasting should not be considered a measure of success of the successful treatment, says Dr. Buchinger.

Exercise and Fasting
Energy, mental acuity, and speed are not faculties directly enhanced by eating. In fact immediately after a meal a person feels sluggish and not at all like being active. Mountain climbers never eat before a climb.

Ask yourself the questions: At which time of the day am I most active? When did I eat last before that time? How much did I eat? Did I have stimulants like coffee or tea then? There is every reason to expect a normal or even better than normal energy level during a fast. I exercise every day throughout my own fast. Almost all fasting experts agree that if you are physically fit, there is no reason that a regular exercise program or sports activity cannot continue during a juice fast. It will help to eliminate toxins and tone recuperating cells and tissues.

Digestive Disorders
Dr. Buchinger, M.D., states[12] that constipation is the most widespread cause of digestive diseases. He explains that doctors often find that their patients pay no particular attention to the fact that they are often constipated. Many consider a daily laxative as perfectly normal compensation. Others find it normal to have a bowel movement only every two or three days. Dr. Bircher-Benner, M.D., the famous Swiss health reformer, points out[13] that one

ought to have a spontaneous bowel movement three times a day! Dr. Buchinger[14] also makes this perfectly clear by reminding us that we usually "take in" three times a day and that we therefore should "put out" three times a day in order to balance the two. It is easy to comprehend then why a large number of diseases have their origin in the bowels. He states in particular certain kinds of headaches, rheumatism, heart and kidney complaints and even the dreaded disease, cancer. In Arabic the bowels are referred to as the *"father of afflictions."* The resultant degeneration of the vital healthy bacterial intestinal flora, a condition associated with deteriorating bowel function, aggravates the problem of poor digestion. Abnormal fermentation and internal decomposition of food residue often lead to problematic flatulence, colic and oppressed breathing. The dire epilogue is not just poor health, but has spill-over effects on the mental state, leading to feelings of gloom and doom. These in turn wreak all kinds of havoc on our lives, from arguments to accidents, and even to suicide. Rather morbidly these are often the tragic outcome of the cumulative effects of improper elimination.

Fighting digestion-originated diseases with pharmaceuticals often enough results in a cover-up. Short term relief is afforded but the problem is frequently compounded. Strong drugs tend to destroy the last remnants of a healthy digestive tract and kill off what beneficial bacteria remain. According to Dr. Buchinger, the best way to repair the bowel is to supplement the intestinal flora, improve eating habits, and undertake a juice fast! He also advocates juice fasting for the treatment of bronchial asthma. Even for allergic asthma he recommends a course of fasting in conjunction with psychological therapy and deep breathing exercises in fresh air.

Kidney and urinary tract diseases are greatly relieved

by juice fasting. To quote Dr. Buchinger, "the fasting person's urine heals its own passages."[15] During fasting the body is enabled to crystallize and shed gravel and even stones. Healthful restoration of similar gall-bladder obstructions is also attributed to juice fasting. However, he recommends a naturopath's supervision during treatment to ease the passing of stones.

For Dr. Buchinger, relief from ulcers does not indicate a regular fasting treatment. I suffered this very syndrome some years ago while engaged in very stressful work at Toronto International Airport. I developed severe digestive problems, which my physician, using barium and lengthy, dangerous X-ray procedures, analyzed as an infection of the duodenal tract with no visible ulcer craters.

Employing orthodox hospital treatment, he put me on a "bland" diet of bananas, milk and cheese, a strong "suppressive" drug containing belladonna, as well as an anti-acid medication. Later I found out that belladonna is a potent poison and anti-acids became habit-forming. It didn't do my digestive troubles much good, and eventually I discontinued treatment.

But how could I be assured of preventing serious ulceration? To begin with, I started supplementing my intestinal flora with Lactobacillus Acidophilus. That helped a little. Then I realized that to effect lasting healing I would also need to change my dietary habits. I started to consciously work on changing my way of eating, favoring fresh fruit and vegetables, and leaving out aggravating foods from my diet, such as carbonated drinks, animal fats and junk foods. I also made some major adjustments to my lifestyle, undertaking regular exercise and a search for less stressful employment. The positive healing that resulted from my combined body and mind approach was simply astonishing. My digestive disorders disappeared rapidly and I've felt fine ever since.

Feminine troubles like hemorrhages, pains, swellings, menstrual irregularities, the change of life, disturbances of menstruation, benign uterine tumors (myoma), which my overweight mother suffered from, can all be alleviated by fasting according to Dr. Buchinger[16].

With other fasting experts, he also recommends the regenerative treatment of fasting for favorable results in chronic poisoning, including those derived from misuse of medications or the use of tobacco and alcohol. Dr. Buchinger holds that afflictions like nervous migraine and chronic headaches, neuralgia, neuritis, chronic insomnia and even hysteria and similar nervous disturbances are greatly reduced by juice fasting.

He states[17] that "fasting stimulates the conductor of the great orchestra of the glands and glandular organs. Those glands which are overactive are toned down and others which act sluggish are stimulated. In short, following the powerful law of compensation in fasting, the organism strives to reharmonize its hormone economy."

Excessive Mucus & The Common Cold

Professor Arnold Ehret was one of the greatest pioneers of healthful living and preventive medicine. His books, especially "The Mucusless Diet," remain bestsellers to this day. In his view[18], biologically wrong, *"unnatural"* foods cause disease which becomes evident through surplus mucus secretion, and in more advanced stages through the secretion of pus, which is, of course, decomposed blood or dead white corpuscles. Fasting will rid the body of excess illness-causing mucus that has accumulated and frequently hardened in the body since childhood. This mucus will then be shed through the urine and excrement. He points to the sticky mucus deposits on the tongue of the fasting person as evidence of this elimination process. The fact that the body suffers from and tries to eliminate excess mucus is even more apparent during a cold, actually an eliminatory process the body uses to rid itself of disease-causing overabundant mucus. Early man, suggests Ehret, lived in a tropical environment, exclusively, and biologically correctly, on fruit. Prof. Ehret[19] recommends favoring mucus-free fresh fruit following a fast, in order to avoid a renewed buildup of surplus mucus. He stresses the eating of fruit for those people suffering from diseases that disallow a fasting period for medical reasons.

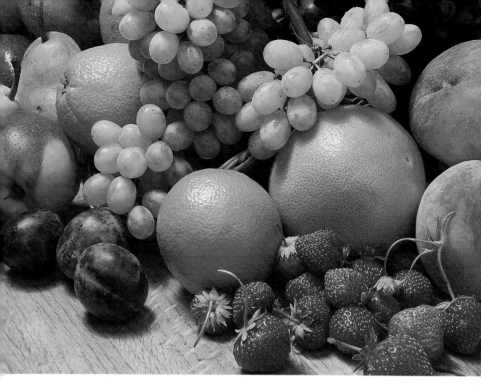

Only quality organically-grown freshly picked, ripened fruits or vegetables assure maximum vital nutrients and freedom from toxins; a *must* particularly during juice fasting.

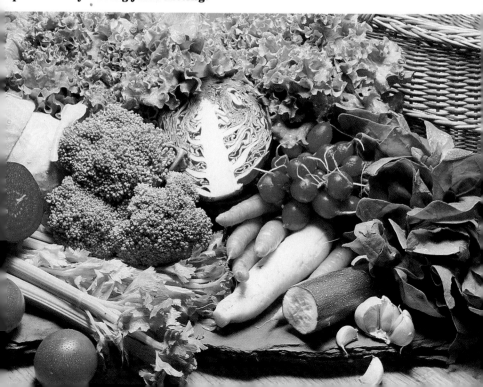

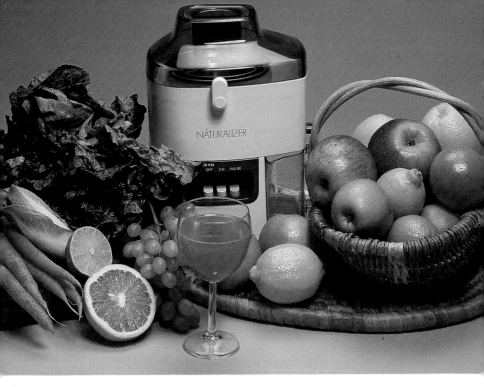

There's a good variety of electrically operated juicers available in most health food stores. These are simple to use and easy to rinse clean.

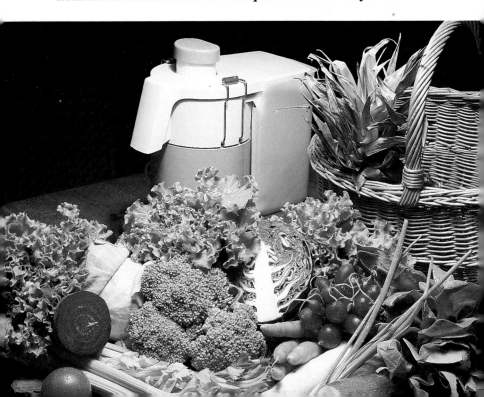

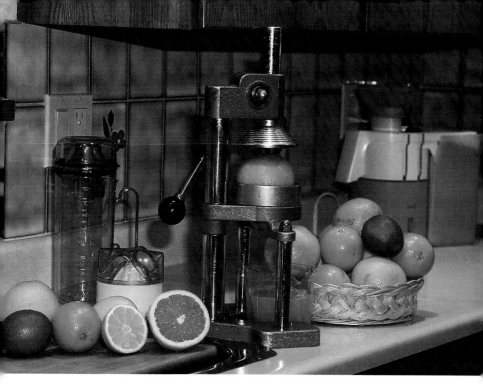

Hand operated juicers come in a variety of sizes and costs.
A light meal idea for your preparation day—fried Tempeh
with Yogurt/Garlic sauce.

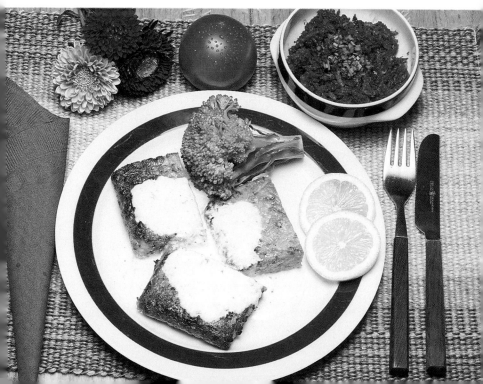

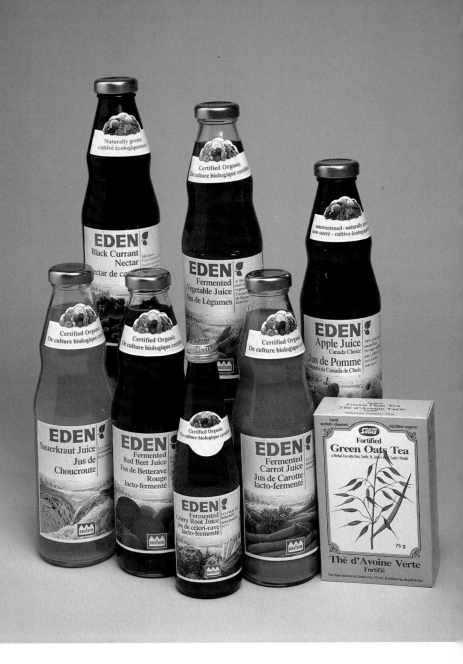

Bottled freshness from pure, organically-grown EDEN juices make juice fasting joyful and effortless.

3

Justifying Juice Fasting

Consider the savings involved in juice fasting. Just a couple of dollars a day will be your total investment for a bottle of juice. From that point of view, juice fasting is more than justified. It's a bargain. Since you will not have to purchase food items during the fast, the money you **save** will be quite considerable.

But how **safe** is it to juice fast?

There is no need to fast for forty days and nights. However, even if you did, chances are you would walk away much healthier than ever. While the body requires a constant supply of liquids (juices), it can live without food for months. However, overeating can kill in a few weeks. There is a vast difference between *voluntary* juice fasting and "being starved to death."

The threats, fear and tortures that accompany most serious ailments can cause severe depression in an afflicted person, creating a greater strain on health than the mere deprivation of food. In fact, it makes all the difference. When you freely choose to fast, you do it joyfully, confidently and with full understanding; free of fear, trauma or problems. I am, of course, referring to a person who is basically healthy.

If you suffer from a serious condition, such as cancer, diabetes, or heart disease, you must be under your physicians care at all times. Still it's up to you to suggest juice fasting to your doctor; he may not have thought of it. Even though juice fasting of up to two weeks poses no danger, I suggest you consult your physician if you feel you do not possess the necessary understanding of all the phases of juice fasting.

Where to Fast?

The answer to the question of where to fast is: Wherever you feel most comfortable. It can be at your home, at work, at the holiday cottage, while visiting friends during a vacation or on your boat. A place you can relax, participate in your favorite sport or follow a hobby, is ideal.

When to Fast?

You can undertake a juice fast at any time. There is no need to interrupt your routine. On the other hand, you may wish to practice your first juice fast during a one week holiday. It's probably a good idea to start on a weekend and carry through to the next one.

How to Fast?

It's advisable to develop a plan for your juice fast. Selecting the beginning of a weekend or similar period during which you will have a couple of days away from your regular job is helpful. Informing members of your household in advance of your fast will give them an opportunity to get used to the idea — they may even join you! It is equally important to tell *yourself* that you are going on a fast. If you tell yourself this a few days ahead, several times every day, the message will reach your subconscious and be transmitted to every cell of your body, thereby better preparing yourself. If the body cells expect to fast, they are anticipating the opportunity to divest themselves of useless material.

A complete day-by-day practical approach to fasting is given from chapters 7 through 11. Prerequisite to a successful fast is exercising control over the body. A resolute mind won't succumb to the rumblings of the stomach. If you refuse to pay attention and are firm in your resolve the rumblings will soon stop.

How Long to Fast?

How long to fast is a very good question. The answer is not often simple. A lot depends on the individual, his or her constitution and aim in fasting. The planned number of days can always be shortened or lengthened in accordance with personal requirements. Generally speaking, if you merely wish to lose weight, cleanse, regenerate and rejuvenate your body, six to twelve fasting days should suffice. I take a short fast such as this once or twice a year. For the beginner six fasting days are optimal.

Then again, maybe the answer could be simply to fast for as long as you feel comfortable with it. Even a twenty-four hour juice fast will have a tonic effect on the system. You might be a person who wants to fast just twenty-four hours once a week. Keep in mind though that the entire length of your alimentary canal measures thirty feet or so from mouth to anus and it'll take longer than twenty-four hours to cleanse your intestines completely, not to mention the other organs and tissues. The more often you fast, the longer you can tolerate a fast. As with everything else, expertise comes with experience.

As for fasting for therapeutic purposes, I would like to quote Dr. Buchinger again: "The more stubbornly chronic and the more anchored in the constitution the disease is, the longer the fast should last."[20] Stretches of up to forty days or even longer should not be undertaken without the strict supervision of a qualified practitioner. You'll have no trouble convincing a naturopathic physician that you wish to alleviate an ailment by means of a controlled fast.

Fasting And Bad Breath

During the first fast there is a tendency to develop a thickly coated tongue and bad breath. The reason for this is simply that the body has hidden the putrefying toxic materials deep within the bowels and cells and is finally given a chance to expel them. Fasting relieves the system of unwanted body odours and bad breath; after a successful fast your breath will be sweeter than ever before. To offset bad breath during fasting, sips of natural lemon juice will help, as will herbs. Once you have cleansed your system through a juice fast, unpleasant body odours will automatically disappear.

Fasting and Smoking

I strongly advise against smoking. If you are a smoker, at least quit for the duration of your juice fast. Tar and nicotine will cause even more harm during fasting than at other times. Once you are on the juice fast, the desire for smoking will diminish and it won't be so hard to do without tobacco. If you smoke and want to quit you may find juice fasting an excellent method for giving up smoking permanently.

Fasting And Enemas

Some may feel like taking an enema every day during a fast. Generally, enemas should be taken only occasionally because they tend to make the bowel sluggish. Waste materials accumulated in the body can cause suffering to the fasting person and enemas can be helpful for avoiding toxin-buildup in the lower bowel during a fast. When the normal bowel action is absent, enemas can assist during a fast by washing out all the toxic wastes from the lower digestive tract. During a juice fast, there is little, if any, elimination because the natural peristaltic motions of the alimentary canal that propel food to its evacuation point is halted. Your bowels' evacuation reflex is not triggered during a fast because *juice is absorbed in the upper intestinal tract*. Juice fasting is such a magical healing measure it will do you good even if you decide not to use enemas during your fast. Regular bowel action will resume automatically with the return to solid food.

I take an exploratory enema after the first day of fasting if there has been no natural evacuation. If much fecal matter is discharged, I take another the following day. If, however, little is eliminated with the warm water, I refrain for the next 3 days. Then, if there still has been no natural evacuation, I test the lower bowels again.

Some precautions for enema use: Make sure the water you use is warm, slightly above body temperature. Always keep your enema equipment clean and disinfected.

Why Juice And Not Water?
A total fast, with just drinking water and no food of any kind, is the most commonly practiced fasting method. But it is not necessarily the best. Freshly made vegetable or fruit juices are rich in vitamins, minerals, trace elements and enzymes. These essential nutrients suspended in juice are easily assimilated directly into the bloodstream with no strain on the digestive system. They help rather than hinder the process of autolysis, or self-digestion, wherein the body consumes its surplus weight. Properly prepared vegetable and fruit juices do not cause the manufacture and secretion of hydrochloric acid in your stomach, which is caused mainly by a diet of solid, protein-rich food.

Raw juices supply an alkaline surplus to your body that is very crucial for proper acid-alkaline balance in your blood and tissues, since blood and tissues contain large amounts of acid during fasting. In the theories of Dr. Ralph Bircher[21], raw juices contain an as yet unidentified factor which stimulates micro-electric tension in the body and is responsible for the cells' ability to absorb nutrients from the blood stream and effectively excrete metabolic waste.

Dr. Ragnar Berg, a Swedish scientist, reputed to be the world's first great authority on nutrition and biochemistry, is quoted as having said: "During fasting the body burns up and excretes huge amounts of accumulated wastes. We can help this cleansing process by drinking alkaline juices instead of water while fasting. I have supervised many fasts and made extensive tests of fasting patients, and I am convinced that drinking alkaline-forming fruit and vegetable juices, instead of water, during fasting will increase the healing effect of fasting. Elimination of uric acid and other inorganic acids will be accelerated. And sugars in juices will strengthen the heart. . . Juice fasting is, therefore, the best form of fasting."[22]

4

Which Juice to Choose?

Raw juices are best when freshly squeezed. With a juicer you can press juices at home or you can buy bottled juices at your health food store. If you do, make sure that these are pressed from completely fresh and organically grown fruits and vegetables, harvested at the peak of their medicinal content. Two good brands are Eden juices or Schoenenberger juices. These will keep indefinitely if left unopened in their original bottles. Once opened they will last up to two weeks stored in the refrigerator. You should not take juices that have been reconstituted from concentrates under any circumstances. They undergo a heat process which eliminates all beneficial enzymes.

Though we own an extractor, we decided, in planning our juice fast, that to purchase fresh vegetables in the variety and quantity we needed was not advisable, simply because store-bought vegetables are not likely to have been organically grown, have probably been sprayed with insecticides or have been waxed. We were unable, as well, to find the right blend of organically grown vegetables. If you do decide to press and prepare your own juice for your fast, carefully scrub all fruits and vegetables with warm water and rinse them several times with cold water. Of course, you are best off if you have your own garden and grow your own fruits and vegetables organically, with the exception that you are restricted to do your fast when fruits and vegetables are in season. Prepare only as much juice as you will need for each day to avoid spoilage. (The results of our own juice fast are described in chapter 6.)

We found the juice we wanted in our health food store. For our own fast, we decided on a lactic acid fermented Eden vegetable cocktail. We chose Eden Sauerkraut juice for our preparation day because sauerkraut juice has a tremendous cleansing and laxative effect. Freshness of Eden juices is guaranteed by the expiry date printed on each bottle.

Lactic Acid Fermentation and Fasting

Some of the Eden juices are lactic acid fermented juices.[23] This process has a protective and healing effect while simultaneously improving flavour. During lactic acid fermentation, acetylcholine is formed — a substance that stimulates the peristaltic movement of the intestines, always an excellent aid to fasting. Lactic acid also tones the nerves, thereby calming the mind and improving sleep. Other substances such as vitamin C and B_{12} are formed, as well as various enzymes. Also generated in this process is choline, which improves, regulates, and balances the composition of the blood, providing it with nutrients. Choline regenerates tired blood and tends to normalize blood pressure. Lactic acid fermentation also produces a substance called glucokinin which is similar to insulin in reducing the blood sugar level. Lactic acid fermentation also reduces the sugar content of the juice itself which is excellent news for diabetics and the elderly. Best of all, it plays a role in preventing fatty deposits, invariably a great help during a fast.

Lactic acid fermentation increases the potassium content of raw vegetable juice, complementing the sodium content through the potassium/calcium/magnesium complex.

Lactic acid fermentation stabilizes the raw vegetable juice naturally, so very little heat is needed. Low heat pasteurization prevents heat damage.

Lactic acid has a bactericidal effect on undesirable intestinal bacteria, allowing those necessary for digestion to operate more effectively.

The well-known Swiss scientist, Dr. Johannes Kuhl, (M.D., Ph.D.), who undertook extensive research on lactic acid fermentation, ascribed a cancer-preventive role to L(+) lactic acid fermentation. Dr. Kuhl suggested[24] supplementing modern cancer therapy with lactic acid therapy. For readers wishing to find out more about lactic acid and cancer therapy, the book "How to Fight Cancer & Win" by William L. Fischer, published by Alive Books is recommended. It must be the Canadian edition, Chapter IX "The Healing Power of Lactic Acid."

Vitamins, Minerals, Trace Elements and Enzymes

The following list of juices is compiled to assist selection of particular juices for particular juice fasting purposes.

The addition of freshly pressed, unrefined linseed oil (flaxseed oil) or unrefined sunflower oil to the juices will aid in absorption of provitamin A, while providing essential fatty acids of the Omega family. Many important enzymes are present in raw juices, but enzymes are rendered inactive by heat over sixty degrees Celsius (Centigrade).

Dr. Georg Lanyi, M.D. states that colouring substances are present in large quantities in juices. These increase production of red blood corpuscles, influence digestive and assimilative processes, and contribute to the metabolism of proteins and cholesterol. In addition, raw juices contain hormone-like substances and antibiotic substances.

*** In the following section juices marked with 3
asterisks contain L(+) lactic acid

Green Oats Tea — Salus

Fortified Green Oats Tea is the herbal tea best suited to
supplement juice fasting because it induces toxic waste
elimination, while strengthening the nerves due to its high
content of trigonelline, saponin, and chlorophyll. The tea
is especially beneficial in therapeutic juice fasting and for
preventing and eliminating kidney stones. It promotes the
elimination of uric acid, supports water elimination from
the tissues, and strengthens the connective tissue due to its
silicic acid content. It is highly recommended in conjunction with the lemon juice and maple syrup juice fast
described below. Salus Green Oats Tea is fortified with
Stinging Nettle, St. Johnswort and Lady's Mantle herbs.

Elderberry Juice — Eden

Elderberry juice is particularly good for a weight reduction fast during the colder seasons, fall, winter and
spring. Elderberry juice aids blood cleansing and is an
expectorant and laxative. It helps rid the body of infected
mucous membranes thereby allaying colds, coughs, and
hoarseness. It alleviates breathing difficulties due to
colds. Elderberry juice has a high concentration of vitamin A and C as well as containing vitamins B_1, B_2, niacin
and B_6. It also contains protein, fat, carbohydrates, sodium, calcium, potassium, phosphorus, iron. If contemplating an elderberry juice fast, feel free to write to me in care
of my publisher for free recipes. Also available from your
health food store or Alive Books is the book "Elderberry
Internal Cleansing" by Dr. Morton Walker.

Lemon Juice + Maple Syrup

Lemon juice, because it is rich in vitamin C content is par-

ticularly beneficial in the spring time when vitamin C
deficiencies are greatest, says E. Schneider, M.D.[25].
According to the Viennese urologist, Professor Dr.
Bibus[26], citric acid in lemon juice is effective in the pain-
less dissolution of kidney stones. Contrary to popular
belief, citrus juices do not cause hyperacidity. In combina-
tion with maple syrup they make an ideal drink for
weight reduction and cleansing. Take note that supple-
mentation with the vitamin B-complex is recommended
when undertaking this juice fast. Two tablespoons lemon
juice are mixed with 2 tablespoons Canada Grade AA
fancy quality maple syrup and a dash of cayenne pepper
is added along with a cup of water. Drink as much of the
mixture as you like during the fast. A word of caution:
Maple syrup consists of 68% pure maple sugar. It is not
suitable for use by diabetics.

Vegetable Cocktail***— Eden
Eden juice cocktail is prepared from selected organically
grown fresh vegetables stock, rich in vitamins and minerals. (We chose this juice cocktail for our own juice fast —
see chapter 6.) Eden vegetable cocktail contains tomatoes,
carrots, red beets, celery, sauerkraut, beans, cucumbers,
cauliflower, silver onions and green peppers. The ingredients are partially L(+)-lactic-acid fermented so that the
biological value of this vegetable composition is boosted,
while its spicy flavour is enhanced. A pinch of pure sea
salt is added to harmonize and round off the taste.

Black Currant Juice — Eden
This sugarless juice contains 1600 to 2000 mg of vitamin
C, as well as 264 mg potassium per kg. It is similar in its
effects to red currant juice (see below). Its tannic acid and
black colouring matter are considered beneficial in treating diarrhea. Those who suffer from this affliction can

include the juice in their regular diet. It should also be considered for the prevention of colds and influenza when it is drunk hot. When fever is present, black currant juice can serve as a refreshing cool drink. Black currant juice stimulates the appetites of those recuperating from sickness.

Eden Red Currant Juice — Eden
This is another prepared sugarless fruit juice high in vitamin C and minerals. Red currant, because of its high potassium and low sodium content, is the only berry fruit permitted in Dr. Gerson's anti-cancer diet. Dr. Gerson advocates[27] just this kind of high potassium and low sodium intake for his cancer patients. This juice, with 2820 mg per kg (mg%), is also high in citric acid.

Blueberry Juice — Eden
The sugarless juice of blueberries grown in the wild is possessed of great healing powers according to Ernst Schneider, M.D.[28] The high content of tannic acid it releases in the intestines has a tonic effect on the bowels and prevents bacterial infection by inhibiting the fermentation-causing escherichia coli bacteria present there. Dr. Schneider advises a three-day wild blueberry fast as a means of freeing children as well as adults from intestinal roundworm and pinworm.

Red Beet Juice***— Eden
In the view of P. G. Seeger, M.D.[29], Head Physician for more than 35 years at the famous "Charite" Cancer Research Department in Berlin, lactic acid-fermented red beet juice is particularly indicated as supportive juice therapy in the prevention of malignancies. He states that red beet juice is a beneficial influence in normalizing cellular respiration of tumor cells. Hans Armin v. Schweinitz

reports[30] animal experiments with rats and mice in which tumor growth was delayed and reduced with the juice. Various researchers have confirmed its positive effect on malignancy prevention and treatment. Eden bottles an excellent red beet juice.

Carrot Juice***— Eden

This juice is available with or without lactic acid. E. Schneider, M.D.[31], states that carotene is transformed in the liver into vitamin A which has a therapeutic effect on tired eyes and prevents night blindness. Carotene suspended in juice is more easily assimilated. Hence a carrot juice fast is particularly helpful for people wishing to improve their vision.

Celery Root Juice***— Eden

Dr. Seeger, M.D., states that the ethereal oil in celery root juice has the effect on the kidneys of increasing urine and caution is indicated in patients suffering acute kidney disease. Because of its stimulating effect on the production of urine, the oil is helpful in circulatory disorders, rheumatism and the prevention of stone formation. It also stimulates the glands. Due to its relatively high carbohydrate content it is unsuitable for diabetics. Ernst Schneider, M.D.[32], recommends celery root juice to eliminate toxic metabolic waste products and mentions its alleviating effect on gout and rheumatism, nervous debility and depression. Otto Gessner[33] also mentions the juice's positive effect on heartburn and acid indigestion. This Eden juice is also partially (L+) lactic acid fermented.

Sauerkraut Juice***— Eden

Partially (L+) lactic acid fermented raw sauerkraut juice is recommended by Professor Kemkes, M.D.[34], of the University of Giessen, Germany for its nurturing effect on the intestinal flora. He also attributes a stimulating effect on the bowels, helpful in chronic constipation, to sauerkraut juice. He considers it a gentle and natural laxative.

Recently Prof. Dr. A. I. Vertanen of Helsinki[35] discovered biologically active substances in cabbage, the source of sauerkraut juice, that inhibit hyperfunction of the thyroid gland. The American physician Carnett Cheney, M.D.[36], published several scientific papers about the treatment of stomach ulcers and duodenal ulcers with raw cabbage juice, claiming that heat application destroys the effective substance.

5

Juiceful Rejuvenation

Youthful Count of the Years

Otto Buchinger, M.D., one of the world's foremost authorities on fasting, says with regard to aging: "Does the cause of aging lie with the impregnation even of the tiniest branches of the blood vessels with calcium and fat-like substances, which make the vessels rigid, narrow, brittle and inelastic, with the cessation of sex-hormone production, or with the enzymes having become increasingly incapable of functioning?"[37]

Many decades ago Professor Ehret emphatically recommended fasting for rejuvenation and agelessness, calling aging a latent disease that can be successfully prevented. He stated that graying and becoming bald, the most striking symptoms of growing old, are caused internally and can be blamed on accumulated toxic mucus which can be eliminated with fruit or vegetable juice fasting followed by adopting healthful eating habits.[38]

Today, geriatric researchers know beyond doubt that all the symptoms of old age are caused by disorders, impurities and faulty performance of the vital nervous system, especially those nerves that take charge of the digestion. In this system that directs all involuntary functions in the body is found the predisposition for growing old. The saturation of the tissues with metabolic poisons is, of course, to be held responsible, along with damage to the body's system from other prevalent poisons such as environmental pollution and tobacco smoke.

My youthful appearance amazes people all the time. Once a salesman visited my office. In conversation he told me that he was 47 years old. He looked it. When we talked about our mutual past, I observed how as a boy in post-war Germany, I often went hungry because there was not much food available. When I recounted certain events from my past he looked at me quizzically and then interrupted, "You can't know these things! How old are you?" It created an embarrassing moment. I told him, "I'm 47." "I can't believe it," he said, "you look twenty years younger than I, and we're the same age!" He shook his head in disbelief, then added, "That's incredible." I usually anticipate disbelief or surprise so I tend to avoid the topic of age. While visiting my brother's family I was racing through the park with my 15 year old nephew. His mother was watching us. She commented to my brother who is three years my senior, "Look at your brother — he is so much younger-looking than you." My brother did not answer and for once someone else was embarrassed.

The secret to youthfulness is simple. I'm a fussy eater. I carefully select the food I put into my body. Few items qualify. As a child I was a terrible nuisance to my mother — I wouldn't eat half of the foods she put on the table. Today, I don't overeat and I fast when I'm not feeling well. I always keep body and mind active. I refuse to look forward to retirement. I grew up in a low country and had never been on skis. Now I live in Vancouver, B.C., and three years ago I took up downhill skiing. A lot of people suggested, "Aren't you too old to learn skiing?" On the contrary, I love downhill skiing and my wife and I are regular visitors at Whistler Ski Village each winter.

A life insurance salesman who wanted to sell me a policy was told, "You can't insure my life — only I can do that." I have never purchased life *insurance* — I would rather practice life *"assurance."* Believe me, it works.

I tell you all this for only one reason — to convince you that staying young for a longer period of time is possible. Mine is not an isolated case; I am just concerned about my health and well-being. Nor do I feel particularly blessed genetically, either physically or mentally. I have 3 older brothers. Each looks his age and has a history of various ailments. Our mother lost her ten-year battle with cancer. Most of her life she had been overweight; she didn't believe in fasting. She thought vegetarians strange. She suffered many illnesses even before her cancer, yet I have almost never been seriously ill. The only time I was ever cut by a doctor's knife was at nine years old. A bee had stung me and its stinger was lodged too deep to be merely pulled out.

The worst sickness I ever had was tick fever, a viral disease I contracted in Africa after being bitten by an infected tick. It kept me delirious for a week, but I emerged just as healthy, perhaps healthier. I believe that a fever can be curative and restorative, ridding the body of toxins, in much the way fasting does. As a point of interest, I did not eat during my tick fever sickness, though I drank.

A song goes through my mind. "I'm gonna live forever, I'm gonna learn how to fly." Fasting is the magic key that opens the door to agelessness. Believe it — you can turn the clock around and look and feel younger. Juice fasting offers a new lease on life. Nature's law of the survival of the fittest is unchangeable, yet there is every reason to rejoice. It is in your power to recreate your body and make it fit again.

Being youthful longer, more beautifully, is only a distant dream for most people. My advice is to rise up against aging and vote for youthfulness. People don't die of old age, but of disease, whether they are young or old. Those who banish disease from their lives through regular juice fasting, healthful nutrition, a positive mental attitude and regular exercise (a form of *"recreation"*) will find so much joy in their lives, they will want to live forever.

Limited effort gets put into continuing to live when there is an inordinate amount of pain and suffering, especially in the later years. But staying young and living long doesn't have to be just a dream. After an eight day juice fast you will feel revitalized and younger.

In Just Eight Days

You can feel as good as new — go for it! An eight day juice fast can restore much of the vitality every human being should rightfully feel most of the time, regardless of age. Here is the simple "magic formula," with details to follow:

One preparatory day — for a first cleansing of your bowels.

Six fasting days — this period will elevate your body to an improved level of metabolism.

One break fast day — this is mandatory to avoid a too sudden return to your regular diet. It guarantees a smooth transition for your metabolism.

Here are some more pointers to help you during a fast:

1. Staying power, the strength to maintain and not resign your fast, is at its lowest during the first three days. During this period you may find it more difficult to stick to your resolution to fast. After this has been successfully bridged

though, your body will be accustomed to the 'all clear' signal and make compensatory metabolic adjustments.

2. Fasting is easier if family or friends join in. Temptations that arise from sitting at the dinner table next to full plates when your own is empty, disappear. If no one is joining you in fasting, it's best that you are not present during their meals.

3. To prevent setbacks (there will be many tempting moments during the first three days referred to as the fasting crisis) you will need diversions. Working at your regular place of employment is one of the best diversions possible. If you are at home, busy yourself with a hobby. Keep your mind on the task at hand. The more intense your work or hobby, the less will you be subject to relapses from fasting.

4. The short eight day fasting treatment does not affect your constitution, because it is less concerned with the reduction of fat than with the cleansing and evacuation of accumulated toxins.

You will require:

- The recommended food on day 1 for preparing your metabolism

- A supply of juice for six fasting days

- The recommended food on day eight to break your fast

to maintain congruity and accuracy, make sure that during the fasting period you weigh yourself without clothing in the morning, after going to the toilet but before showering, and before drinking your juice.

6

The Day-By-Day Miracle Vegetable Cocktail Juice Fast

When my wife, Gabriele, heard of my plan to write a book about juice fasting, she suggested that it would give readers greater insight if I presented an authentic report on an actual fast and offered to be the guinea pig. She decided to fast on a vegetable juice cocktail made by Eden, and came back from the health food store with enough Eden vegetable cocktails for an eight day fast.

While researching background material on juice fasting, it occurred to me that I, too, could lose the extra pounds girding my waist and stomach, while deriving benefits from a cleansing of my metabolism. One look in the mirror persuaded me that I was "upholstered" in the wrong places and would go further without my "spare tire." I nearly went on a lemon juice fast, then opted to follow Gabriele's lead, reasoning that two identical accounts are more convincing than one.

We discovered that fasting together is even more fun than fasting alone. We had a dinner engagement on the first Saturday in July, so we chose Sunday to launch our juice fast. Cancelling all further dinner invitations, we informed our friends that we were going on a "juice fasting holiday".

I trust you will find the following account of our fast illuminating as well as instructive. It is copied directly from my diary and, I hope, will further encourage readers who are currently contemplating a juice fast.

Preparatory Day

Sunday morning. We get out of bed and record our weights:

Gabriele 150.0 lbs. Klaus 174.5 lbs

We are both tall. I measure 182 cm (6'2") and Gabriele 171cm (5'7"). I am 6.5 lbs overweight and my wife 15 lbs. over her ideal weight.

After our morning exercise we each drink a glass of sauerkraut juice made from lactic acid-fermented white cabbage. It tastes refreshingly zesty, not sour, as I had anticipated. The purifying action of the sauerkraut juice is producing swift results.

We enjoy a delicious breakfast. (prepared in accordance with the meal plan in chapter 7) Lunch and dinner are easily prepared and turn out to be delightful meals. Toward evening I develop a headache. I know that my system has accumulated plenty of pernicious toxins that "yell" at my brain, demanding reinforcement. Obviously I have been indulging in undesirable foods far too often. This time I have no intention of heeding the noxious call. I instinctively know that this is a curative headache and constitutes the first crisis point for my resolution. I haven't had coffee or tea for at least twenty-four hour. The headache is most likely caused by caffeine withdrawal.

I drink a cup of malva herb tea and relax to watch a film. Any absorbing diversion or activity will alleviate early fasting crisis symptoms and avert any possible desire to discontinue a new fast. Tea and a stirring show are the right remedy for me. My headache vanishes.

Gabriele is feeling fine, sitting at her Singer in the next

room, stitching a new dress. She has extra time to indulge in her favourite hobby during the fast as she doesn't have to cook.

First Fasting Day, Monday

Weights: Gabriele 149.0 lbs. Klaus 173.0 lbs.

At our morning weigh-in, Gabriele comments with amazement that she has already lost a pound during the preparation diet. We have EDEN vegetable cocktail juice for breakfast. We decide on drinking non-carbonated mineral water to combat thirst throughout the juice fast.

Around 5:00 p.m. Gabriele returns from an intense day at the office complaining of a mild headache and sensitized stomach. It seems to me that her accumulated toxins are being consumed and are fighting back. She sips a cup of hot lemon balm tea, has a relaxing interlude, and soon both of her upsets are miraculously gone. Diversion, it is clear, is the key when starting out on a cleansing vacation. I spend my extra spare time, completing a water colour painting I had started some time before.

Second Fasting Day, Tuesday

Weights: Gabriele 147.0 lbs. Klaus 172.0 lbs.

Who says you don't lose weight the first three days?

Gabriele is down 3 pounds and I've lost 2.5 lbs. We feel good on waking and throughout the day. I have the first bowel movement this day since beginning the fast. When not fasting I have at least one every day. Obviously my system is determined to hang on to every available nutrient for as long as possible.

Third Fasting Day, Wednesday

Weights: Gabriele 145.0 lbs. Klaus 171.0 lbs.

Getting up slowly is good advice during a fast. Sit on the edge of the bed for a moment and stretch, then get up, go to the wash basin and splash cold water in your face. Gabriele has lost 5 lbs! I'm lagging behind having lost only 3 lbs. At my regular half hour workout this morning, I am surprised how strong I feel. I sip my apportioned vegetable cocktails throughout the day instead of guzzling them down at the appointed times. Some variation won't hurt. Both of us feel great with no more headaches or feeling of hunger.

Fourth Fasting Day, Thursday

Weights: Gabriele 143.0 lbs. Klaus 170.5 lbs.

It does cross our minds several times to indulge while riding our bikes along English Bay but we don't let ourselves be tempted by the aromas drifting from the food vendors at the Sea Festival.

We begin taking enemas to assist the cleansing process. With no solid waste to eliminate, the bowels, too, have a vacation. Losing two lbs. daily is a great satisfaction to Gabriele. My losses slow to a half-pound per day. Women accumulate water more easily than men and her vanishing pounds are mainly water and toxins.

The time spent in preparing and eating five meals a day is now at our disposal. It serves as a welcome opportunity to catch up on reading.

My urine turns to a muddy yellow. It had been clear before this — a sure sign of toxins leaving my body! Paul Bragg, N.D. Ph.D., the prominent fasting expert, explains that the cloud in the urine consists of unwanted mucus that must be eliminated for the body to be truly healthy.[39]

Gabriele turns our juice cocktail into a delicious-tasting warm soup, adding 2 tbsp of chopped parsley, 1 tsp of chopped chives, 1 dash each of oregano, garlic powder and black pepper. A true gourmet soup!

Fifth Fasting Day, Friday

Weights: Gabriele 142.0 lbs. Klaus 169.0 lbs.

For a change I lost 1.5 lbs and Gabriele only 1 lb on this day. The tides are turning. We exercise as usual and the cocktails still satisfy any feelings of hunger. For the first time, I supplement my juice fast with vitamins (A and D, beta-carotene, B-complex, C, E) and minerals (selenium, silica*, magnesium, garlic)). They can't hurt and don't add weight.

Sixth Fasting Day, Saturday

Weights: Gabriele 141.0 lbs. Klaus 167.5 lbs.

We are still dropping pounds. This is our last fasting day. In the afternoon we go on another bike ride.

Eighth "Break Fast" Day, Sunday

Weights: Gabriele 141.0 lbs. Klaus 165.0 lbs.

I lost another 2.5 lbs. We feel proud and elated. One of our passions is food and this is the very first time that we have gone on a juice fast together. We find our joined effort to be an animating and spiritual experience, shedding unwanted pounds while simultaneously giving new

---

* *To find out why I supplement with silica, I invite you to read my book "Silica — The Forgotten Nutrient." It contains vital data on geriatrics!*

strength to our bodies and even our marriage!

7

Feasting For Your Fast

The preceding chapter told you what we did — now it's your turn.

It is mandatory to prepare for your fast by reducing your food intake at least a day before juice fasting. Choose light foods like low-fat (2%) yogurt, low-fat cottage cheese or quark, fruits and raw vegetables. What is quark? I have been asked that question often. Quark and cottage cheese are the milk solids separated from whey. They are similar, yet not alike. While cottage cheese is made from sweet milk with rennet to make it curdle, quark is made from soured skim milk that curdles naturally. Quark contains valuable lactic acid, while cottage cheese usually contains milk fat and stabilizers. Quark can be found in delicatessens and often in health food stores. It's also easy to make at home. Simply take buttermilk, warm it to approximately 70° Celcius (158°F) for about 15 minutes and pour into sieve or through a cheese cloth. Within hours or overnight you have quark separated from the whey. Skim milk quark has the consistency of cream cheese and can be used for most recipes. If you prefer you can make quark from kefir milk or plain natural yogurt, the one without flavourings, stabilizers or carrageen. Kefir milk and plain yogurt needs to be warmed up in the oven to about 100° Celcius (212°F) for at least one hour. I make my own yogurt with cultures I buy in health food stores. Rosell Institute has yogurt and kefir while Hansens supplies yogurt and an excellent Acidophilus culture. All these come in portion packs enough to make 1 to 2 litres (quarts), while Natren supplies a super yogurt culture in a glass bottle, which makes many batches of excellent yogurt with up to 80% L(+) Lactic acid.

It's a good idea to apply some means of cleansing your bowels, such as drinking several glasses of EDEN L(+) Lactic acid fermented sauerkraut juice. This can be started a few days in advance.

Your First Day

A good recipe for preparedness follows:

Immediately after rising, on an empty stomach, drink a glass of EDEN sauerkraut juice, approx. 200 ml. This juice has a stimulating zesty flavour and will also start off your bowel cleansing.

Your breakfast should consist of a good-tasting cereal (Try Muesli with approx. 266 kcal) but no more than 200 g. Skip coffee, instead have another glass of sauerkraut juice (26 kcal). Avoid eggs, cheese, meat etc. You might want to replace your cereal with a slice of whole wheat bread with some butter and fresh low-fat quark (or cottage cheese) sprinkled with chives.

10 o'clock break should be observed with another 200 ml of sauerkraut juice.

Lunch consists of quark with herbs, which you can prepare in advance as follows: 100 g low fat cottage cheese or quark mixed with 60 g of low fat (2%) yogurt. A sprinkling of sweet fancy paprika, caraway seeds to taste, and a pinch of sea salt — unless you live on a salt-free diet. Add a small to medium onion, finely chopped, and a dash of dill to taste. Fold in 50 ml of regular,stiffly whipped, 30% fat whipping cream. Gives a fresh natural treat and has only 330 kcal. Or cook 40 g of unshelled rice and eat together with 250 g steamed apples or apple sauce. Finish off with a cup of unsweetened camomile tea.

Afternoon break — Again drink 200 ml of sauerkraut juice.

Dinner — 100 g low-fat quark stirred with 50 ml of regular milk and sweetened with honey to taste. Add a few almonds or nuts. This (approx. 450 kcal) will satisfy your hunger during the night and prepare you for the next morning. Or have a slice of whole rye bread, butter and a low-fat cheese on top. How about a cup of peppermint tea just before bedtime?

8

Easy Eight Day Juice Fast

Fasting is fun and will quickly agree with you. The best part is that you no longer need to look at your watch to find out if it's time to eat. Of course, fasting is rarely easy; if it were, everyone would be doing it. It requires dedication to go without food.

To avoid hunger pangs which will only arise during the first two or three days the juice of your choice is taken in seven portions. The EDEN physician recommends to drink:

150 ml at 8:00 am	150 ml at 5:00 pm
125 ml at 10.00 am	125 ml at 7:00 pm
150 ml at noon	150 ml at bedtime
125 ml at 3:00 pm	

That adds up to 925 ml of home-made juice (or one EDEN bottle of 750 ml + 225 ml from the next bottle). In this way you will overcome any desire for solid food. In three days you will have drunk 2,775 ml of juice (or used up approx. four EDEN bottles) yet will have ingested only 292 kcal daily. That approximates 10% of your regular fare depending on individual eating habits, of course, so you can imagine how intensely your body now draws on its fat reserves while eliminating accumulated surplus body fluids, together with metabolic waste and toxins.

Don't let yourself get thirsty during these three days. Drink as much calorie-free liquid as you require ie., mineral water, or fruit teas without sugar. The herbal tea I highly recommend is Fortified Green Oats Tea made by Salus-Haus in Germany with green oats, nettle, St. Johnswort, and Lady's Mantle. This tea is alkaline, provides iron and other minerals, is a perfect blood cleanser and keeps you calm. Avoid any liquids that might aggravate your stomach or nerves such as coffee or black tea during your fast.

The juice included, you should take in about three litres of fluid each day. Fluids without calories act like an internal body rinse, flushing your system, rather than being retained by your tissues.

To add spice and variety to your fasting life, here are a few "permissible" variations:

- Adding a crushed garlic clove and a smidgen of sea salt or "spike" to vegetable juices. To eliminate garlic odour, simply add some freshly chopped parsley. A few drops of peppermint oil will also do.

- Spicing it with 1 tsp grated orange peel, but only from chemically clean oranges!

- 1 tsp grated ginger or ginger powder and some honey

- 2 tsp grated horse radish, a dash of sea salt and a zip of lemon juice

- 1 tsp curry together with one quarter grated apple

- 2 tsp fresh tarragon

- 1 tsp of lovage, a European herb of the parsley family

- 3 tsp chopped watercress and a dash of sea salt
- 1 tsp of freshly minced sage used sparingly!

These are only suggestions and should stimulate you sufficiently to give wings to your own flights of fancy. Fasting is nowhere near as boring as you might have imagined.

There is variety galore. Other ingredients you may try are lemon juice, caraway seed, basil, mugwort, savory, dill and dill seed, chervil, chives, parsley, rosemary, celery seed and salt, ground cloves, coriander, nutmeg, pimento, soy sauce and, yes, mushroom powder.

Your Loss is Your Gain

The phrase sounds like a paradox, but isn't. You will have gained in many ways, most notably in increased well-being. While some of the more intricate metabolic benefits now happening inside your body could only be ascertained through a lab analysis, this is quite unnecessary. You alone are entitled to measure your most obvious success. With the help of your bathroom scale you can check some of the changes happening inside your body — and add to the fun and excitement. If you own a blood pressure gauge, you will also find improvements in blood pressure levels.

Use the following table to control your daily progress:

Your weight in the morning of the preparation day:

_____lbs_____kg

Observations:_____

Your morning weight on the first fasting day:

_____lbs_____kg

Observations:_____

Your morning weight on the second fasting day:

_____lb_____kg

Observations:_____

Your morning weight on the third fasting day:

_____lbs_____kg

Observations:_____

Your morning weight on the fifth fasting day:

_____lbs_____kg

Observations:_____

Your morning weight on the sixth fasting day:

_____lbs_____kg

Observations:_____

This is your last fasting day, **UNLESS** you decided that real happiness is found in the <u>Intensive Fast</u>, or <u>Two By Six Day Fast</u> with one day break in between. If so, my heartfelt congratulations and please turn to chapter 9 for further instructions regarding the **VIBRANT FOUR-TEEN DAY JUICE FAST.**

Your morning weight on the breaking fast day:

_____lbs_____kg

Observations:_____

---

to maintain congruity and accuracy, make sure that during the fasting period you weigh yourself without clothing in the morning, after going to the toilet but before showering, and before drinking your juice.

9

Interlude
For A Two By Six Day
Juice Fast

How to Proceed During Your Interlude Day

During your previous six fasting days your body obtained only 60 g of protein. To compensate, your interlude day prescribes a protein-richer, but still light fare. Use this day well. It puts your metabolism into a changed position from which it can easily switch to juice fasting again. So please eat only in accordance with these recipes on this day. You will then take in only 964 kcal while supplying your body with 84 g protein, an amount which will suffice beyond this day. By the way, this interlude has no noticeable influence on your fasting results.

You may, if you wish, change the sequence of these meals, as long as you keep to the total calorie count, however, start with a particularly rich protein meal.

Recipes for the Interlude Day
In the morning:

Chocolate Cream — Mix 100 g low-fat quark (or cottage cheese) with 2 tbsp (20 g) de-oiled cocoa powder. Add 3 tbsp of 10% cereal cream, then strain. Mix in 2 tbsp of a select honey and fold in a stiffly beaten egg white. This delectable dainty has 406 kcal and 27.3 g protein.

At lunch:

Quark Piquant — Mix 100 g low-fat quark (or cottage cheese) with 1 small jar of capers (and one half of the caper liquid). Add 1 medium-sized chopped onion (40 g) and spice with a dash of white pepper from your pepper mill, 1 tbsp freshly chopped parsley and 1 tsp chopped caraway. This satisfies your appetite. It contains 112 kcal and delivers 18 g protein to your system.

Afternoon break:

Savory Austrian Jelly — Also known as Colourful Aspic. In a glass bowl, blend 1 cup (200g) lactic acid-fermented homemade (or try the EDEN brand) sauerkraut, 2 sticks (50g) finely chopped, raw celery shredded, 2 tbsp diced red peppers and 1 medium-sized diced (40 g) onion. Mix altogether with 1 tbsp freshly chopped parsley. Dissolve a little pectin in 100 ml hot, but not boiling, apple juice. Pour the solution over the sauerkraut mixture and put into the refrigerator for a few hours. Tastes great and has only 158 kcal and 9 g protein.

At dinner: before 8:00 p.m.

Tribute from Emmenthal — Put 75 g low-fat quark (or cottage cheese) through a strainer and mix with 5 g finely grated 45% fat Emmenthal cheese. This must be marked Swiss Emmenthal in red ink, because there are a number of inferior products on the market, simply marked "Swiss" or "Emmenthal", usually in blue ink. These should be avoided as they are made from pasteurized, homogenized milk which does not produce the proper fermentation processes required to achieve Swiss Emmenthal. Add 1 tsp of mild mustard, 1 freshly chopped medium-sized onion (40 g) and 1/2 tbsp sweet paprika. Fold in 1 egg yolk and serve. This gives you another 30 g protein for your next six fasting days, but delivers only 343 kcal to your body.

Following this interlude day, continue with your next six fasting days, as under the eight day fast, ending your fast in the same manner prescribed in the "Your Break Fast Day" section above.

10

Vibrant Fourteen Day Juice Fast

Congratulations to those of you who have decided on the intensive fast. Your perseverance is admirable. Perhaps you have discovered to your own amazement how much previously undiscovered singlemindedness and tenacity you possess; how much stamina and strength you can muster. Perhaps you have merely convinced yourself to continue after the sixth fasting day. You know by now that juice fasting doesn't consist of penance, hapless denial, and mortification of the flesh. Your sixth fasting day is your *interlude day*. This day is used to raise the level of protein in your body. Turn to the Interlude chapter for details.

Health is a gift of nature but won't stay with us throughout life if we don't make a definite effort to sustain it. Some sort of sacrifice is necessary to maintain good health, especially when much of the time we are overeating, eating the wrong foods or even indulging in junk food. A two by six day juice fast is the perfect way to do penance, to give the body a chance to recuperate from all the ill treatment bestowed on it and make it whole again. Your body will thank you by emanating new feelings of youth and freshness. Your scales will confirm your new lighter self and the mirror will show a more beautiful, radiant you. Your inner health will reflect your outer appearance. This will be your greatest reward.

There is more. Your forbearance in fasting is also compensated with a well-defined distinguished success. It is simply astonishing how your metabolic well-being becomes noticeable. Accelerated cell renewal does not take place suddenly during the first six days but the effects increase gradually. After fifteen days you will see very clear ramifications: your skin will surprise you with a refreshed, glowing radiance, proving that true beauty comes from within. The performance of your skin will have intensified. It is now ready for grooming and non-decorative cosmetic application.

Well-being can be further increased by intensive body massages, calisthenics and other exercises — even a simple walk through forest or park will reflect heightened beauty and awareness.

Unless you decided to make your own juice, you will need another eight bottles of vegetable or fruit juice or cocktail, making a total of seventeen bottles for the two by six day fast. Crisis points may arise again during your continued fast. Always remember that they are rarely of long duration and will in almost all cases pass by themselves, leaving you in control. Should unanticipated problems not pass within a reasonable time, you should consult your naturopathic physician or doctor immediately before continuing to fast.

You may want to augment your juice fast with vitamin and mineral supplements. Your naturopath or nutritionally oriented physician and health food store can help you choose the right supplements.

If you are unable to receive proper advice, I suggest to take a complete multi-vitamin with chelated minerals, the one I prefer is Dr. Duenner Super 2, two tablets per day. Better still is the liquid multi-vitamin Epresat from Salus-Haus. Also, three capsules of Efamol Oil of Evening Primrose, for the daily essential fatty acid supply.

Optional to the above are one or two capsules A and D, 400 I.E. Vitamin E (the most natural form being d-alpha and mixed tocopherols) Natural Factors or Dr. Duenner, as well as Vitamin C up to 500 mg daily. If you have a tendency to being anemic I suggest to take Floradix herbal iron tonic daily, as recommended, which also provides B Vitamins and Folic Acid. Use the following table to continue control of your daily progress of your *second* six day period:

Your weight in the morning of your intermission day:

_____lbs_____kg

Observations:_____

Your morning weight on the seventh fasting day:

_____lbs_____kg

Observations:_____

Your morning weight on the eighth fasting day:

_____lbs_____kg

Observations:_____

Your morning weight on the ninth fasting day:

_____lbs_____kg

Observations:_____

Your morning weight on the tenth fasting day:

_____lbs_____kg

Observations:_____

Your morning weight on the eleventh day:

_____lbs_____kg

Observations:_____

Your morning weight on the twelfth and last fasting day:

_____lbs_____kg

Observations:_____

Your morning weight on the breaking fast day:

_____lbs_____kg

Observations:_____

Eight Exits for Toxins

There are eight bodily exits for toxins. We have seen how marvelous cleansing juice fasting is, and how poisons are eliminated from the body during a fast in a number of ways:

1. Via the bowels. While eating solid food your bowels are busy digesting; during a fast they are only eliminating and resting.

2. Via the skin. Don't be concerned if your skin doesn't smell good while you are fasting. The pores are finally open and eliminating. Frequent washing or bathing is advisable during a fast. To prevent dryness use a good natural skin care cream, but don't plug up your pores with make up during your fast.

3. Via the lungs. Exhaled breath is loaded with metabolic waste residue in gaseous form. Do deep breathing exercises in the fresh air or at an open window. Turn your heat off at night and sleep with at least one window open. Bad breath during a fast is a good sign that the lungs are eliminating toxins.

4. Via the mucus membranes — Nose, throat and wind pipe mucus self-cleansing is increased during fasting.

5. Via the mouth. Observe the surface of the tongue. It will be covered according to the level of toxicity in your body. Use your tooth brush on the tongue and rinse the mouth with water as much as required. To eliminate bad odour ingest some fresh herbs like chives, dill and parsley.

6. Via the urine. At times the urine will darken in colour and smell strong. These are signs that toxins are being expelled. Increase water consumption to flush out your system when the urine darkens or gets opaque.

7. Via the vagina. The mucus membranes of the vagina will also increase cleansing activity during a fast. An increased discharge is temporary for the duration of the fast.

8. Via the mind. This may seem eccentric, but it is true. Don't be afraid of increased dream activity, aggressive thoughts and moods or depressed moments. Speak your mind during your fast. If you are alone, it would be a good idea to write down your feelings and thoughts. You will find that by the end of your fast you will have gotten rid of a lot of *mental waste*.

11

Break Fast At Breakfast

Breaking your fast correctly is extremely vital to the success of your juice fast. According to Dr. Otto H. F. Buchinger, "even a fool can fast, but only a wise man knows how to break the fast properly and to build up properly after the fast!"[40]

The most important rule for breaking your fast is: Do not overeat! Allow several days of light eating to gradually readjust your metabolism to your regular food intake. Start off with easily digestible foods like fruit, raw vegetables, or yogurt with a few nuts. On the second day, add a light soup or vegetable salad for dinner. On your third day, you can try a slice of bread with butter and cheese. Thereafter, you can probably return to your regular diet. If you have fasted longer than 10 days, prolong the breaking-in period by one day for each four days of additional fasting. Keep in mind not to overeat. In fact, you may wish to keep this in mind permanently. It is the foremost rule for maintaining a healthy body and for looking, feeling and acting young at heart.

Return to Solid Food
Congratulate yourself on having made it — almost. The fast breaking day is a necessary "bridge" and should be strictly adhered to (in accordance with the suggestions listed below) in order to assure the full benefit to your

system, and to avoid stomach upsets.

These foods will return your body slowly and gently to solid food. Your metabolism that has concentrated on within, must get accustomed again to obtaining its nourishment from *without* — in other words — from your regular diet.

Recipes for Breaking Your Fast
(Eight day and two by six day fasts)

In the morning:
Fruit quark: Thoroughly mix 75 g low-fat quark (or cottage cheese) with 2 egg yolks and 2 tbsp (50 g) honey. Gently steam 100 g fruit (peach, apricot, Syrian (yellow) plum) with 1 tsp lemon juice and 1 tbsp honey. Dissolve a little pectin into the fruit mixture. Mix the still warm fruit with the quark, let cool and enjoy. This delicacy amounts to 482 kcal, but delivers only 11.6 g fat to your now sensitive metabolism.

Lunch:
Potato soup: Take 4 medium-sized potatoes (300 g), 1 carrot (60 g), 1 celery root (30 g) and a handful of leek and dice into 1/2 litre of regular milk (3.5%) and simmer until very soft. (Caution: Burns easily, so be sure to simmer) When ready, pass through a strainer and serve with freshly chopped chervil. A filling meal with only 577 kcal however it burdens your metabolism with only 18.3 g fat.

Or for 2 people:
Rice cookies with spring sauce: Cook 1 cup (130 g) of rice in 1 cup of water with a pinch of sea salt. Stir 2 eggs and 50 g finely grated Gouda cheese (45% fat) into the still warm rice. Add a dash of nutmeg and let cool a little. Meanwhile create the spring sauce by dicing 1 large tomato

(100 g), and stirring the finely diced pieces into 75 g low-fat quark together with 1 tsp tomato paste and freshly chopped chives (30 g, about 1 bunch). Use a table spoon to scoop out small portions of the rice into a frying pan, flatten to small cookies and fry golden-brown on both sides. (Use only 20 g butter for frying!) Serve the warm cookies together with the spring sauce. That adds up to 1,089 kcal and 43.1 g fat, or per serving 545 kcal and 21.5 g fat.

Afternoon break:
Strawberry milk (for 2): Use a fork to mash 150 g strawberries. Add 2 tbsp honey and the juice of half a lemon. Mix into 300 ml low-fat milk (2%) (Stir the mashed fruit into the milk, not the other way around.). Cool lightly and serve. Amounts to 362 kcal and 5.5% fat, or 181 kcal and 2.75 g fat per serving.

Dinner:
Apple quark: Take 75 g low-fat quark and 4 tbsp buttermilk, 2 tbsp whipping cream (30% fat), 1 tbsp lemon juice, 1 tbsp grated horse radish and mix thoroughly. Take 1 medium-sized apple (150 g), grate, then stir into the quark. Makes a zesty tasting meal that yields only 329 kcal and 14.7 g fat.

Or:
Simple Muesli: Take 50 g oat flakes, 1 tbsp honey and 125 ml regular milk. Yields 322 kcal and 5.3 g fat.

Even when you choose the most fattening of the above recipes, you will hardly exceed 50.35 g total fat intake. Choosing the lowest fat dishes, you will reach only 37.75 g fat.

These meals assure that your metabolism is gently returned to "normal." The average adult, undertaking a normal daily work load, requires approximately 70 g fat daily in his/her normal diet. To impress upon you the necessity of your fast, consider that the average fat consumption is around 140 g daily. That amount is too high!

12

Broken Fast

Don't feel too badly about a broken fast. If you didn't stick with it, that's alright. There is always time to try again. Broken fasts are fairly common. There are many reasons for them and no need to chide yourself. Instead pat yourself on the shoulder for having tried. An initial failure can stimulate a second try and strengthen the resolve in the long run.

Keeping The Faith

For those who kept the faith and did stick to a planned fasting schedule, no doubt it was a fun experience for you and a much-needed recuperation period for your body. It is a good idea to repeat a juice fast once or twice a year. The second attempt will be even easier than the first, and a repeat performance brings other advantages. Your body is being taught to live on smaller meals and this will last for some time, until out of forgetfulness you start to burden your metabolism again with larger portions. But don't let it go that far. Before these old, deleterious ways return to wreak havoc on your figure and your internal well-being, introduce a repeat juice fast.

Keeping to this pattern, you will be gently led to improved, "nutri-physiologically" superior eating habits. Your future will be free of any feelings of deprivation, renunciation or sacrifice. The beneficial effects of your changed lifestyle will increase from year to year with advancing age.

Next time you may want to try a different juice. If you like the EDEN juices, try EDEN Red Beet Juice with the nutritiously valuable L(+)-lactic acid, which has a toning effect on your metabolism. Or try EDEN Carrot Juice, with pro-vitamin A from which your body manufactures vitamin A, excellent for stomach and intestines, good for your eyes and skin. Or try the interesting EDEN Celery Juice, filled with minerals and trace elements important for hair and bones. Sample the certified organic Vegetable Juice, ready-mix liquid following a well-tested recipe that contains a mixture of valuable and vital nutrients. These will all be available at your health food store.

13

Spiritual Rejoicing

You are tremendously wealthy, hold a dream job and own a beautiful home? That is wonderful and certainly worthy of achievement. But are you happy? You may discover areas in your life where you are either too rich or too poor. How's your health? Without radiant health even the richest person can feel poor. Health is the first prerequisite to happiness. With juice fasting health can be retained and perhaps even restored to those who have lost it. Juice fasting not only cleanses, regenerates and rejuvenates your body, but also has a profound stimulating effect on your mental faculties. It increases spiritual awareness, mental acuity, and puts you in touch with yourself and the world.

It is imperative to adopt a relaxed attitude, both during juice fasting and afterwards. You will be more sure of yourself, even improve your posture. Try to disassociate yourself from your usual everyday problems. Rest, exercise, read a good book and meditate while juice fasting, and you will create renewed vigor for your body, your mind, and your spirit.

Nature will look more magnificent then ever after a fast. Life will take on new meaning. You will count your blessings, not your problems. You will be amazed how previously unknown positive thoughts and new ideas will arise to stimulate you to renewed vigour. A juice fast will recharge, renew and rejuvenate your whole personality — inner and outer, body, mind and spirit.

That's what it did for us. We are planning our next rejuvenating juice fast for the fall — using elderberry juice to ward off the threat of catching a cold during the winter months.

For every feast there should be a fitting fast. Follow this rule, cultivate a healthful lifestyle, and undertake a juice fast now and then. You may find yourself fasten on joy every day of your life.

The Beginning . . .

References

Trinken Sie sich jung mit mir!
Karin Tietze-Ludwig, Eden, 1988

How To Keep Slim, Healthy And Young With Juice Fasting
Dr. Paavo Airola, Health Plus Publishers, 1971

Holunder-Saft-Kur
Vis Vitalis Zechelius, 1986

Die Zitronensaftkur
K. A. Beyer, Edition AUM, 1985

Die Ahornsirup-Zitronensaft-Kur
Verlag Natur & Gesundheit

The Miracle Of Fasting
Paul C. Bragg, N.D., Ph.D, Health Science, 1988

About Fasting
A Royal Road To Healing
Otto H. F. Buchinger, M.D., Thorsons Publishers Limited

**Die gesundheitlichen Wirkungen der Gemuese
und Fruchtsaefte**
Biopress Verlag

Heilfasten
Helga Duerselen, ECON Taschenbuch Verlag, 1986

**Rational Fasting for Physical, Mental
and Spiritual Rejuvenation**
Prof. Arnold Ehret, Ehret Literature Publishing Co., Inc., 1987

Health and Happiness Through Fasting
Fred S. Hirsch, Ehret Literature Publishing Co., Inc, 1987

Wie neugeboren durch Fasten
Dr. med. H. Luetzner, Graefe und Unzer Verlag

How to Fight Cancer & Win
William F. Fischer, Alive Books, 1988

Index

Endnotes

1. The Bible, King James Version (Fasting - abstaining from physical nourishment): 1 Sam. 1:7, Grief: 2 Sam. 12:16, Anxiety: Dan. 6:18-20, Ps. 69:10

2. Prof. Dr. Zabel, Werner, Germany

3. Selye, Hans, M.D., Canada, The Stress of Life, Stress Without Distress

4. Edison, Thomas A., U.S.A.

5. Dr. Buchinger, Otto H. F., M.D., About Fasting, A Royal Road to Healing, Thorsons Publishers Ltd., Wellingborough, Northamptonshire, England, 1983

6. Breuss, Rudolph, Advice for the prevention and natural treatment of numerous diseases - CANCER - Leukaemia and other seemingly incurable diseases., Rudolf Breuss Publishers, Bludenz, Austria, 1982, p. 44

7. Franklin, Benjamin, U.S.A. American president & inventor

8. Dr. Airola, Paavo, N.D., Ph.D., Juice Fasting, Health Plus Publishers, Phoenix, Arizona, U.S.A.

9. EDEN Doctor: Der Saft-Fastenplan von Eden, p. 2

10. Dr. Buchinger, Otto H. F., M.D., Germany, loc cit

11. Dr. Buchinger, Otto H. F., M.D., Germany, ibid

12. Dr. Buchinger, Otto H. F., M.D., Germany, ibid

13. Dr. Bircher-Benner, M.D., Switzerland, Bircher-Benner Handbuch, Bircher-Benner-Verlag, Gmbh, Bad Homburg v.d.H., Germany

14. Dr. Buchinger, Otto H. F., M.D., Germany, loc cit

15. Dr. Buchinger, Otto H. F., M.D., Germany, ibid

16. Dr. Buchinger, Otto H. F., M.D., Germany, ibid

17. Dr. Buchinger, Otto H. F., M.D., Germany, ibid

18. Prof. Ehret, Arnold, Rational Fasting, Ehret Literature Publishing Co., Inc., Dobbs Ferry, N.Y., U.S.A., 1987, p.

19. Prof. Ehret, Arnold, The Mucusless Diet, ibid

20. Dr. Buchinger, Otto H. F., M.D., Germany, loc cit

21. Dr. Bircher, Ralph, M.D., Bircher-Benner Handbuch, loc cit

22. Dr. Berg, Ragnar, Nutritionist/Biochemist

23. For technical information on lactic acid fermented juices and other EDEN products, readers may write to: Eden Waren, Bad Soden - Taunus West Germany or Flora Distributors Ltd. Box 67333 - Vancouver, BC

24. Dr. Kuhl, Johannes, M.D., Ph.D., Checkmate to Cancer

(Schach dem Krebs)

25. Dr. Schneider, E., M.D., Düsseldorf
26. Prof. Dr. Bibus, Urologist, Vienna, Austria
27. Max Gerson, M,D., A Cancer Therapy, Gerson Institute, Bonita, CA, 1958, p. 227
28. Schneider, Ernst, M.D.
29. Dr. Seeger, P. G.
30. von Schweinitz, Hans Armin
31. Schneider, Ernst, M.D., loc cit
32. Schneider, Ernst, M.D., ibid
33. Gessner, Otto
34. Prof. Kemkes, M.D., University of Giessen, Germany
35. Prof. Dr. Vertanen, A. I., Helsinki, Finland
36. Cheney, Carnett, M.D., U.S.A.
37. Dr. Buchinger, Otto H. F., M.D., loc cit
38. Prof. Ehret, Arnold, loc cit
39. Bragg, Paul C., N.D., Ph.D., The Miracle of Fasting, Health Science, Santa Barbara, Ca., U.S.A., 1988, p. 188
40. Dr. Buchinger, Otto, loc cit

Suggested Reading

Diet, Nutrition and Cancer
Committee of Diet, Nutrition, and Cancer, Assembly of Life Sciences, National Research Council, National Academy Press, Washington, DC 20418

Drink Your Troubles Away
John Lust, Benedict Lust Publications, New York, NY, 1975

Fasting • The Buchinger Method
Maria Wilhelm-Buchinger, the C.W. Daniel Company Ltd., Saffron Walden, England, 1984

Fresh Vegetable and Fruit Juices — What's missing in your body?
N.W. Walker, D.Sc., Norwalk Press, Prescott, AZ, 1978

How to Get Well
Paavo Airola, Ph.D., N.D., Health Plus Publishers, Phoenix, AZ, 1987

How to Keep Slim, Healthy and Young with Juice Fasting — the Age-old Way to a New You!
Dr. Paavo Airola, Ph.D., N.D., Health Plus Publishers, Sherwood OR, 1971

Make Your Juicer Your Drug Store
Dr. L. Newman, Benedict Lust Publications, New York, NY 1970

The Bristol Detox Diet For Cancer Patients
Alec Forbes, M.D., Keats Publishing, Inc., New Canaan, CT, 1985

Traditional Foods are Your Best Medicine
Ronald F. Schmid, N.P., Ocean View Publications, Stratford, CT, 1987

The Complete Raw Juice Therapy
Thorsons Editorial Board, Thorsons Publishers Limited, Wellingborough, England, 1977

Books Published
by

Devil's Claw Root and
Other Natural Remedies for Arthritis
Rachel Carston, Alive Books, Vancouver, Canada, 1985, 125 pp

Fats and Oils
The Complete Guide to Fats and Oils in Health and Nutrition,
Udo Erasmus, Alive Books, Vancouver, BC, Canada 1987, 363 pp

How to Fight Cancer and Win
William L. Fischer, Alive Books, Vancouver, BC, Canada, 1988,
287 pp

Kitchen Guide to Fats and Oils
Siegfried Gursche, Alive Books, Vancouver, Canada, 1990, 56 pp

Making Sauerkraut and Pickled
Vegetables at Home
Annelies Schoeneck,
Alive Books, Vancouver, Canada, 1988, 80 pp

Silica — The Forgotten Nutrient
Klaus Kaufmann, Trophologist, Alive Books,
Vancouver, Canada, 1990, 108 pp

Marvelous Melbrosia — The Key to
Fertility and Virility
Rhody Lake, Alive Books, Vancouver, Canada, 1990, 56 pp

Self Help Guides

by

A popular series of small booklets, 24-48 pages each presenting a variety of topics with well-researched and reliable information.

Acne — Donald Howland, M.D.

Arthritis — Donald Howland, M.D.

Basic Guide to Nutrition & Health — Maurice Benner, M.D.

Breast Disease — Maurice Benner, M.D.

Devil's Claw — Hildegard Pickles

Evening Primrose Oil — Maurice Benner, M.D.

Green Gold — Wheat & Barley Grass Juices — The Nutritional Treasures of the 20th Century — Sonya Bass

Heart Attack & High Cholesterol — Donald Howland, M.D.

Help Your Heart — Ernst D. Kuehl, M.D.

How I Cured Myself of Cancer — A Testimony of Howard N. Wagar

Hyperactivity — Donald Howland, M.D.

Menstrual Problems — Donald Howland, M.D.

Multiple Sclerosis — Donald Howland, M.D.

Nutrition and Aging — Maurice Benner, M.D.

Obesity — Donald Howland, M.D.

Schizophrenia — Donald Howland, M.D.

Vitamin A — Maurice Benner, M.D.

Vitamin B_3 — Maurice Benner, M.D.

Vitamin B_6 — Maurice Benner, M.D.

Vitamin C — Maurice Benner, M.D.

Vitamin E — Maurice Benner, M.D.

Zinc — Maurice Benner, M.D.

Alive Self Help Guides are available in Health Food Stores attractively priced at $1.95 to $4.95

Focus On Nutrition

is an in-depth newsletter filled with vital information on a variety of current health topics. These pamphlets are available at Health Food Stores at a suggested retail price of 35 cents, or by subscription from Alive at $1.00 per copy. You will find the information in these newsletters most interesting and thought-provoking. The topics are chosen carefully and, covering a variety of nutritional themes, present well-researched and reliable information in concise form.

1   The Hot Potato: Food Irradiation — Karen Hanke

2   The Miracle Workers: Golden Linseeds - Flax
        — Karen Hanke

3   Yeast: Facts & Fallacies — Karen Hanke

4   Roots and Bulbs: The Miracle Healers You Should
        Know About — Karen Hanke

5   Thank Goodness for Health Food Stores — Karen Hanke

6   Fighting Fatigue? Iron — Our Most Widespread
        Mineral Deficiency — Karen Hanke

7   Protecting Yourself Against Cancer
        — Paul Gerhard Seeger, MD

8   Garlic — Can it Remove Candida, High Blood Pressure,
        Worms, and Vampires? — Kathleen O'Bannon

9   The Powerful Healing Magic of the Evening Primrose
        — Alan Donald

10   Silica: A Vital Element for Good Health
         — Johannes Schneider, MD

11   Feverfew — Farewell to Migraine and Headaches —
         Karen Hanke

12   Wheatgrass — Green Power for the Body — Rhody Lake

13   The Personal Energy Crisis — Fatigue — and How To
         Overcome It — Kathleen O'Bannon

There is a tremendous demand for these newsletters. Your Health Food Store may not always have all of them on hand. We recommend you subscribe to 'FOCUS ON NUTRITION,' 24 copies for $24.00 includes mailing fees. Your subscription begins with the first issue. You will be mailed current issues every two months, as titles become available. Send orders to:

Alive — Focus on Nutrition
4728 Byrne Road
Burnaby, BC, V5J 3H7
Canada

About The Author

Klaus Kaufmann, trophologist for alive books, is mainly self-taught. Historical events of World War II and the turmoil following denied him the privilege to attend university. Yet his thirst for knowledge was unquenchable. Klaus has been studying the healing properties of the plant world for many years. He started investigating natural science. His fascination with nature grew and took him all over the globe. Following a photo safari to the African continent, he decided to live for three years in Southern Africa. There he obtained first hand knowledge of a healing flora such as the wonderful Fever Tree. He then took his wife to the equatorial reaches spending a year as a teacher in Kuala Lumpur, Malaysia and acquiring intimate knowledge of tropical fruit. During 1977 the Kaufmann's moved to White Rock, BC to participate actively in miniature horsebreeding. Klaus had started the first such horse farm in Canada several years earlier with friends.

At the age of ten, Klaus won a book prize in his native Germany for an outstanding children's story he wrote. After that his interest in writing blossomed alongside his growing interest in all matters related to health. Following the study of English literature and creative writing at university, his professor appointed Klaus editor of *CONTACT*, a Canadian Writers Guild publication. Under his editorship the publication expanded from a simple newsletter to a magazine. When Klaus left, the publication was popular in book shops and read at universities across Canada and in England. Some of Kalus' poetry was selected for a live performance in Toronto, Canada.

According to Klaus, his commitment to the health food movement started in the early Sixties when one day he decided to create a *meatless meat sauce*. Since then he has worked as marketing manager for a Canadian health food manufacturer and, over the years, has written articles and books for alive books. He wrote his enormously popular book, *Silica — The Forgotten Nutrient*, for regeneration and longevity. Klaus' still unfinished mammoth reference work *The Encyclopedia of Natural Healing* nears completion. Books on other health topics are "in the works."